# LL COOL J's
## PLATINUM WORKOUT

# LL COOL J's
## PLATINUM WORKOUT

## LL COOL J

### AND

## DAVE HONIG

#### WITH JEFF O'CONNELL

RODALE

To my family and children

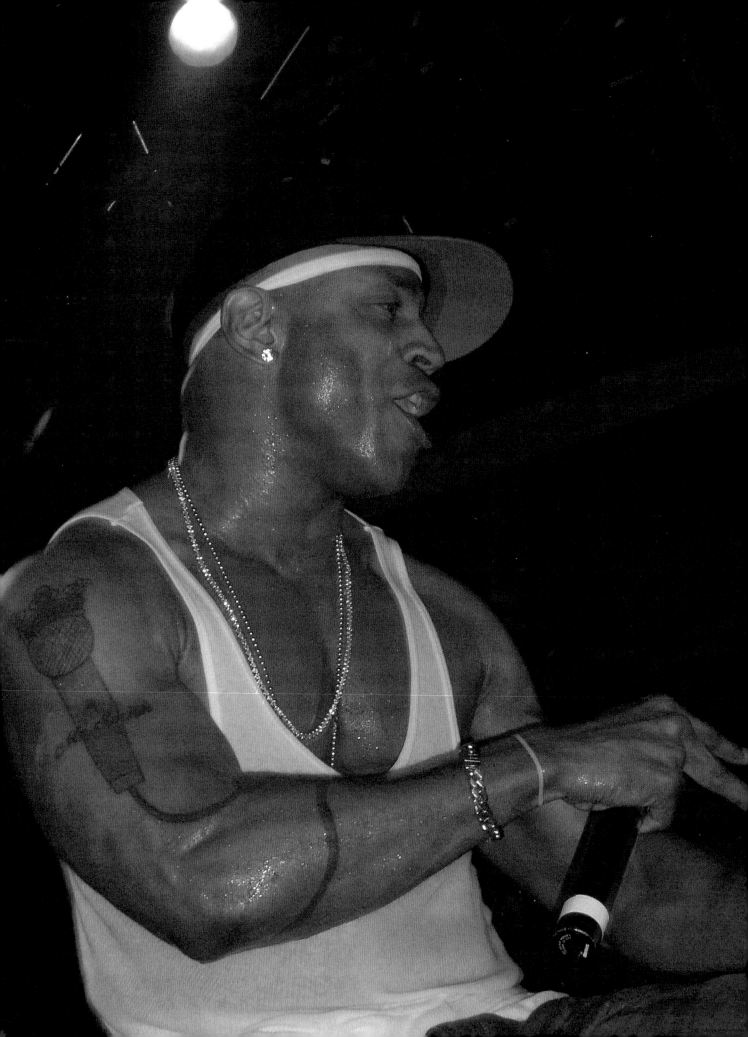

# CONTENTS

# ACKNOWLE

**Thanks to** David "Scooter" Honig; Jeff O'Connell; William Morris Agency; Jonathan Pecarsky; Jason Barrett of Alchemy Entertainment; James and Dennis at Powerhouse Gym in Bayside, New York; Four Seasons Hotel Los Angeles at Beverly Hills; Brian Daughtry; Joan Allen; Michael Hertz; Debbie Smith; Chris Mohr; Jimmy Peña; the entire staff at Rodale Books; Monica Morrow; my good friends focus, determination, and willpower; and my Lord and Savior, Jesus Christ.

—LL COOL J

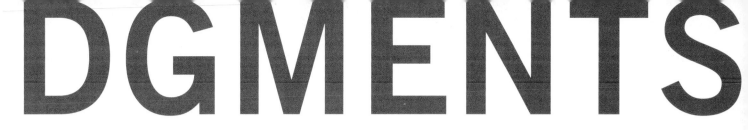

# DGMENTS

**I'd like to thank** James Todd Smith for giving me the opportunity to work with him and be a part of this project; my mother, Frances "Mama Duke" Honig, for her strength and courage; my dad, Michael Honig; my brother, Victor Honig, and his wife, Leslie; Marisa, Michael, and Megan Honig; my niece, Madison Honig, for her perseverance; Debbie Smith, for putting up with this for 24 years and still being normal (all my love); Derrick Panza; Powerhouse Gym of Queens; Reverend Joe Allegro; Chris Aceto; Paul Holtzman; Barry Schneider; Q-Tip; Wyclef Jean; Leonardo DiCaprio; Tyler Perry; Jeff Frankel; Peter Gaudioso; Brian Daughtry, my main man; Donald Gardner; Robert Podowlsky; Dr. Margaret Goodman; Bob Jackson of Gleason's Gym; Steve Ward of Champion Nutrition; Dr. Bob Palazzo; Zab Judah; Vivian "Vicious" Harris; Dmitry Salita; Vinny Maddelone; and Eddie Guyton, for being there for the fight.

—DAVE "SCOOTER" HONIG

**Thanks to** Suliette Baez, Phillip Cassidy and Powder Valley Mill, Cathy Clay, Jeanine Detz, Joe Dowdell, Amel El-Zarou, Marc Gerald at the Agency Group, Chris Lockwood, Rita Madison, Lara McGlashan, Chris Mohr, Peter Moore and David Zinczenko at *Men's Health*, the O'Connells, Jimmy Peña, Liz Perl and Zach Schisgal at Rodale Books, Scooter Pie, Pete Siegel, Veena & Neena, Heidi Volpe, and Zoraida Walker. Special thanks to LL Cool J, Megan Newman, Sherilee Newton, Steven Stiefel, and Joe Weider, the Master Blaster.

—JEFF O'CONNELL

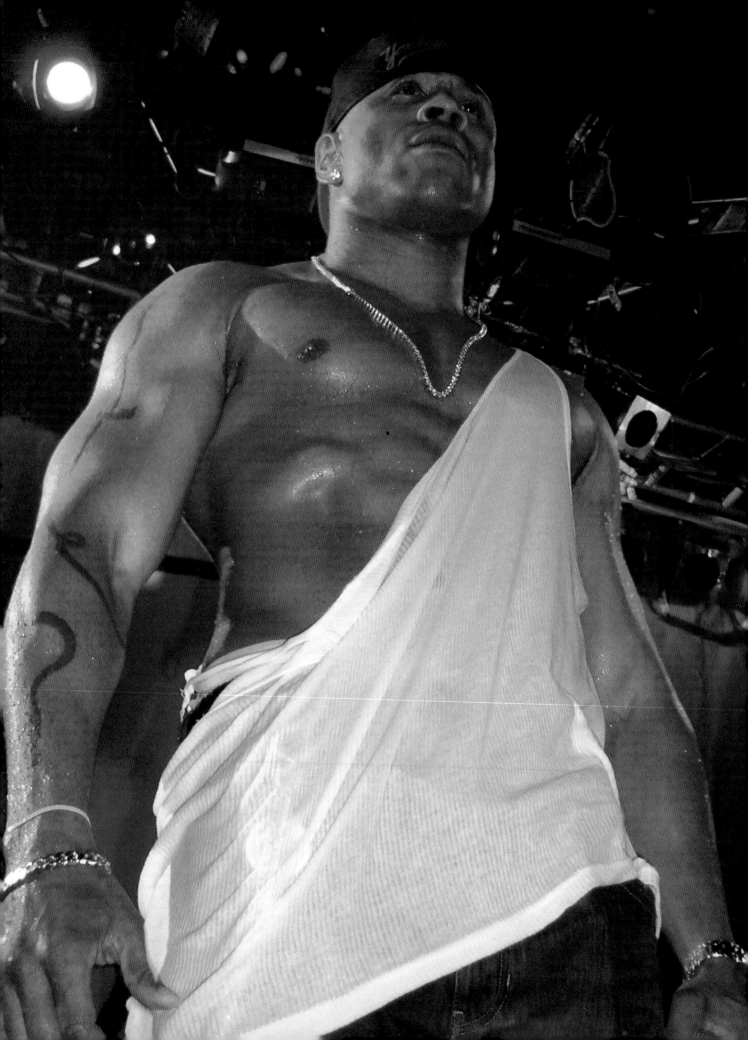

# PREFACE

**W**HEN I first committed myself to writing *Platinum Workout*, I thought, *What are people* demanding *in a fitness book? Forget for a minute about what I want to supply. What are you demanding?* From my perspective, I would think that you would want a book that's truthful, that's honest, that's kind of hard-core, and that's not fluffy. You want the raw.

You want the real deal because one of the biggest decisions that anybody anywhere can ever make in their life is to be the best that they can be. But how many people actually make that decision? I made my decision right after making the movie *Rollerball* and before the *Ten* tour. I was sitting there eating two slices of pizza, one on top of the other, talking to somebody, and I said, "I'm going to lose 40 pounds. I'm done. I've got to do it. I have to take it to the next level. I *have* to."

I achieved that, and it changed my life, both physically and emotionally. ***I want this book to change* your *life, too.*** I want to show you how to achieve *your* own personal version of the platinum body. If Tom Petty goes platinum, he doesn't get an LL Cool J album—he gets his own, right? I'm not just talking about sets and reps; I'm talking about enlightenment; I'm talking about a paradigm shift. That's what I had. Which is why this book is so beautiful: I *know* for a fact that if you follow these workouts and dietary guidance, you'll get where *you* want to go, and your new body will help get you there. ***Success is guaranteed.***

As I write this, my new video, for the song "Control Myself," stands at No. 3 on the Billboard charts. Crazy, isn't it? That's an immensely satisfying accomplishment not only for me as an artist but also for everyone else involved in its creation. To say that it was a team effort would be an epic

> **Either write something worth reading or do something worth writing about.**
>
> **—BENJAMIN FRANKLIN**

understatement. I had a great song that I penned with two coauthors. I had a great producer for the record, Jermaine Dupri, and an equally great director, Hype Williams, working the lens for the video. These are genius-level talents, the best of the best in the world at what they do. I had a one-in-a-million artistic collaborator to challenge me and elevate my game, the amazingly talented Jennifer Lopez. No elaboration required.

But my secret weapon, the thing people talked about everywhere, from hard-core gyms and hair salons to office watercoolers and street corners, was my physique. I don't care if you've got lungs like Pavarotti and dance moves like Fred Astaire or Michael Jackson, you *cannot* pull off that song and that video while trying to suck in a belly. Uh-uh. Ain't happenin'. That's not what I meant by "control myself."

When you're in a video with J. Lo and people talk about your body as much as hers, you have earned the right to say that you've accomplished something significant. But I didn't always look like this. Trust me, I'm not some sort of phenom like Mr. Olympia, Terrell Owens, or Lance Armstrong. If you watch syndicated reruns of my old TV show *In the House*, you'll see for yourself that I haven't always had a diesel body. I wasn't fat, but "cut" was something the director said at the end of a take, not an adjective people used to describe what I looked like. Now and then I would grab a dumbbell or pedal an exercise bike, but I wasn't serious, and I wasn't educated enough about my training to take my God-given genetics and make the most out of them.

That's a really important point to drive home from the start: ***There is nothing inherently unique about my body.*** I'm not some special guy whose amazing, incredible "specialness" made all this possible. No—this was purely a decision supported by a willingness to work hard to accomplish what I needed to accomplish. You know what I'm sayin'? It's important that all of you know that you can do anything if you put your mind to it. That includes achieving the same level of conditioning that I have.

I really took my body to the next level when the time came to hit the road in 2002 in support of my CD *Ten*. Working with my trainer, Dave "Scooter" Honig, I ended up exceeding even my own highest expectations. That's because working together, ***we developed a revolutionary workout system that not only burns away body fat for good but also builds muscle at the same time!*** In fact, the building of the muscle and the burning of the fat simultaneously is what produced the body you saw in "Control Myself." We call it the Platinum Workout, and it's a surefire way to turn those love handles around your waist into bulges in the good places: your chest, shoulders, arms, and legs.

But I'm getting ahead of myself. That's the end result. To get there, Scooter and I take standard lifts using dumbbells and barbells, plyometrics such as ballistic pushups, fighter's moves, calisthenics, endurance training, and more and blend them into what we call our combination platter, just like they have at certain fast-food restaurants, only healthy. If we can't identify the right movement to tax the body a certain way, not to worry: We just invent it ourselves. Trust me, Scooter Pie is what MacGyver would be if that character had been a personal trainer. He could take you into a room right now with a dumbbell and a rubber band, and in no time you'd be gettin' it on and poppin'. You'd be so sore it would take a forklift to get out of bed the next morning.

That's what makes our workouts unique, and the workouts are what make the book unique. It signals an end to the one-size-fits-all routines repeated over and over again in cookie-cutter workout offerings. That's because I bring the same kind of creativity to my workouts that I bring to my art. With me providing the inspiration and Scooter causing the perspiration, you're about to enjoy working out *more* than ever before, even while working out *harder* than ever before, en route to achieving a body you never thought possible in as short as 5 weeks or as many as 22, depending on how far you want to take this. The program is backed by the most cutting-edge science and research available, which you'll see referenced throughout, but we've done the hard part by simplifying things so you know exactly what to do from start to finish. It's all presented in an easy-to-use format anyone can follow. We're not sending anybody to the moon here; we're just taking you to the gym for some amazing workouts.

While the program is always easy to understand, it's not always easy to accomplish. I don't mess around when I train; I blow and go. When you're running between pullups, dips, pulldowns, situps, doing the treadmill in between, and then jumping on it *again* at the end, you *feel* it. *Period.* You know what I'm sayin'? You have to be serious about getting in shape if you want the platinum body. That's because two constants in my approach are (1) maximum intensity and (2) the kind of focus that could bend a spoon like that kid in the first *Matrix*. And that mind-muscle connection is why my new body is just the tip of the iceberg. The real secret is what this workout program has done for the rest of my life, including my career.

So many people out there aren't willing to make the sacrifices necessary to be in the best shape they could possibly be in. As a result, they assume everyone else must be cheating. People often make comments about me like "Oh, he must be doing steroids" or "He must be on some type of drugs."

That's a self-esteem issue—for them. I'll tell you what they're *really* saying: "I don't have the strength and the fortitude and the ability and the wherewithal to endure the pain that it must take to get into *that* kind of shape. Therefore, he had to cheat. Because if he didn't, that means that he's more focused, more determined, more ambitious, and more aggressive than I am, and I can't accept that. So I'd rather say he cheated."

That is such a cop-out. It's like saying the class valedictorian had to have notes written on his shoe, that there's no way someone could have studied all night and skipped sleep and crammed and gone on the Internet and researched everything in order to get those grades. He *had* to cheat. That's unfortunate because people who excel academically really do put in the work, the same way I rock the weights. Before sitting down to write this, I trained for 45 minutes in the gym at the Four Seasons Hotel in Beverly Hills. That may not be remarkable—only I was up at 4:30 this morning, in a car by 5:00, on a plane by 7:00, flew 6½ hours goin' back to Cali, had two important business meetings once I arrived— and *then* did that workout, which had my heart rate racing from beginning to end. And in a few minutes I will head over to *Jimmy Kimmel Live* to perform five songs on national television.

Would I have rather gotten some sleep and bailed on my workout? Are you kidding me? Of course! But the key to this whole thing is doing what you're supposed to do even when you don't necessarily want to. That's discipline, and discipline creates consistency, and consistency breeds success. That 45-minute workout I just did means nothing if it's only done once, but think about how you'd look if you did that every day for 6 months. Just *that*! And just ate halfway decent. So are you willing to put the cake down, the ice cream back in the freezer, and the fast-food burger back from where it came? I've never seen a single person with abs of steel eating a doughnut, have you? ***When you're no longer willing to tolerate what's* in *your life, you can get it* out *of your life.***

Being in shape helps the hustle. It helps everything. It helps you make money, too, because even if you're not in front of the camera, you're sharper, you're more alert . . . you're just better. When I don't work out, I feel guilty because I know I'm not on top of my game.

It's time to get you on top of yours. Congratulations: You've embarked on a journey that's going to change your destiny. I'm glad you're coming with us. It'll be the ride of your life, for your life.

—JAMES TODD SMITH,
BEVERLY HILLS, CALIFORNIA,
APRIL 2006

# chapter one

# THE ROAD TO MY PLATINUM BODY

> Singleness of purpose is one of the chief essentials for success in life no matter what may be one's aim.
> —JOHN D. ROCKEFELLER

**I**'VE BEEN a boxing fan all my life, and while I've never entered the ring for a world championship bout, preparing to go onstage for a rap concert is probably about as close to that feeling as you can achieve. It's that hyped up, you know what I'm sayin'? A crowd eagerly anticipates your arrival, waiting for the first chord or the ding of the bell to unleash its collective energy. The buzz in the air is so thick, you think the venue is plugged into some mysterious energy source. Once onstage or in the ring, you bob and weave, trying to find your flow, burning more calories than Martha Stewart working the dials on her stove. The collective outpouring from the crowd washes over the stage/ring, but you're unaware of it because you're so in the zone. Song leads to song like round to round. You need to stay strong and go the distance—but you always keep your eyes open and look for your opening. I'm gonna knock you out.

This was the tour in support of my comeback album, *Ten*, released in 2002 to both commercial success and critical acclaim. I had worked out for years, but I had accomplished more in the previous 6 months than I had in all those other years combined. Back in the day, it was just pushup contests and hitting the heavy bag and maybe going to the gym once a week, basically to hang with the fellas. No dieting, no nutrition—just a down-and-dirty street style of working out to maintain some kind of conditioning. There was absolutely nothing scientific about it. One day I was looking in the mirror at my body, and I just wasn't happy with what was goin' on. I became fed up with looking at myself that way. If I'm unhappy with something, I don't accept it; I fix it. So **I made the decision right then and there that I was going to do everything I could to achieve the best possible shape of my life**, without even really knowing what that would look like or feel like.

I set my sights on making it happen for this tour. I was determined to take it to the next level, so I asked my personal trainer, Dave "Scooter" Honig, to join the rest of the crew and me on the tour bus. At the time I weighed 223 pounds, and once he was onboard, I told him, "Scooter, I just want to get down to 210 pounds. If we can accomplish that, I'll be ecstatic." Little did I know that we would actually end up building more muscle than I ever dreamed possible, all while burning fat and getting ripped.

Next thing I knew, we were hopping off the tour bus in the middle of the desert in New Mexico, 115 degrees outside, watching our ride drive off without us, the bus blurry in the heat. The driver would pull off the road 5 miles ahead of us and wait for me to catch up. On foot. Hot? The bugs couldn't walk, it was so hot. The turtles were taking a rest. Maybe it was the heat coming up off the asphalt, but it felt like I was running in hot grease, my calves were burning so bad. Still, we would do that

2 days a week on the road because we were spending so much time driving from one venue to another. It wasn't just a matter of getting from here to there either. We would clock ourselves and try to improve each time.

That's the type of dedication that you must have to succeed at this. What's your highway in the desert? Is it working hard all day and then going home to take care of your family before you can even think about picking up a dumbbell? Your tour is your life. Your tour is work, kids, school, trying out for a team, or whatever. It's different for all of us.

For me, it was passing a school, having the driver pull over, and scrambling over the fence for a makeshift workout. I'd run around the track, do pullups off the football goalpost, bang out some pushups in the end zone. It was crazy, wasn't it, Scoots?

Scooter recalls: "We used supersets. We used pre-exhaust sets. We used straight sets. We used circuits. It all depended on what I thought Todd needed to accomplish on that particular day. I incorporated anything and everything in a concerted effort to confuse his muscles.

"We might go from heavy benches to weighted dips and weighted pullups, and then sprint for a minute, followed by stomach crunches. I'd throw intervals into the mix as well. If a treadmill wasn't available, we'd use stepups, or jumping rope, or mountain climbers. That's what we did a lot on the road.

"He has to rock 'n' roll onstage, so the goal was to keep his heart rate elevated during his training sessions. We don't always have to do this, but the goal on that tour was to burn as many calories as possible in the shortest amount of time. I'd also break the workouts up. Sometimes we'd do our runs early in the morning, and then later in the day, once it had cooled down, we would do our weight training."

# Rock Hard

When you're training that intensely, you really need to keep an eye on your diet as well. After walking into a diner at 3:30 one morning, Scooter asked the cook to clean the grill off because he didn't want the grease on the grill entering my body. The guy looked at him, thought he was crazy, took a $5 tip, cleaned the grill, and then cooked for us.

Other times we would stop at a truck stop in the Deep South, those places where they sell anything from guns and flannel shirts to rebel flags. There was a small diner attached to one such truck stop, and here come seven black guys and one little white guy—Scooter—walking in through the door. We sit down and the waitress comes over holding her notepad and missing several teeth.

She goes, "What can I do for you fellas?"

I said, "We'd like to order, please."

She goes, "You've got to wait a minute. I got to go take the money over at the register, and then I've got to just clean those tables."

So she buses the tables, handles the money, washes some glasses. Then, without washing her hands, she comes straight back over to us.

"Okay, now what can I getcha?"

We all look at each other for a few seconds, and then Scooter says, "We'd like to order. Can I please speak to the cook?"

She goes, "You're lookin' at her, honey."

He says, "Well, ma'am, I'm sorry but you're not cooking our food. Take me to the kitchen. Would you mind if I cook?"

She goes, "No."

So Scooter went back there and made us egg-white omelets. All the guys went crazy.

Scooter: "We would stop on the road, the rest of the crew, from the lighting guys down to the bodyguards, and, boy, can they eat. One of the guys on the bus is the rib king. He would always ask the driver to stop at those rib joints that pop up on the side of the road, the ones where you can see the smoke coming out of the windows from a mile down the road. You think fire trucks are coming there, only they're just cooking ribs in a tin barrel. Anyway, this guy had a built-in homing device for those joints, and as soon as we stopped, Todd would look at me, and I would look at him and say, 'You're not eating it.' Every time, the rib king would have a sour stomach."

Even at five-star hotels, Scooter would go in the back and ask the chefs to please cook his way. It was hilarious: At the Four Seasons in Beverly Hills, they had Scooter's Menu on the wall for Mr. Todd Smith. It was crazy.

Scooter: "After the show, whether we trained would depend where we were that day and how long of a ride we'd have to the next town. Because Todd needs to sleep. So I figured, since he's up, and it's 12:30, we'd get a bite to eat, and then we'd get our workout in. That way he'd have more time to sleep. When you're on the road, it's very important for your client to sleep because he's performing and there's a lot

**LL'S MUSCLE-BUILDING TIP** It doesn't really matter *when* you lift during the day—just so long as you lift. Testosterone levels are naturally highest in the morning, which might give you a little more intensity. At night the weights might boost your metabolism at a time when it normally slows down. Either way, these differences are negligible and tend to cancel each other out. Train whenever it best fits your schedule.

# SCOOTER'S *FAT-LOSS TIP*

If you eat until you're full, you've lost the battle. Always leave the dinner table with a desire to consume more food—but the discipline and foresight to get up and leave.

of traveling involved. So what we'd usually do was, he would sleep, get up and eat, we'd train, he'd go back, lie down, relax—and then we'd go to the show. All the meals would be sent to his room.

"That was the easy part. If we were on the bus, we couldn't stop because we had to reach the next gig, no ifs, ands, or buts about it. You have 8 hours to get from Point A to Point B. So I'd have to serve food on the bus. And I would be cooking chicken breasts, smoking up the cabin—the guys would go crazy. I was the king of tuna. Everybody wanted me to make Scooter's Tuna Special for them, with mayo, sliced tomatoes, a little lemon-lime juice, a little pepper, and a little celery. I would mix that all together and make a nice platter—and everybody would enjoy that. That was the Scooter Meal."

## The Man in the Mirror

In the middle of that tour came the moment of truth: We had gotten the single "Luv U Better" heated up on the radio, and it was time to shoot the video. I was doing some barbell rows a day or two before the cameras were to roll, and I looked up at the mirror, and all of a sudden I saw the form. I saw it! I said, "*Yo*, this is *real*." I saw the shape, I saw the cuts, and I was like, "This is crazy." I had never really noticed it before, but all of a sudden, I just saw it. I was like, "Wow—this thing is really working!"

You're probably wondering how I could have sustained such an intense training regimen and gotten in shape for a video in the middle of a concert tour. It sounds crazy, I know. But through years of training fighters and other world-class athletes, Scooter has developed a unique knack for pushing the human body just far enough to make it respond without pushing it over the edge. See, boxers have to build some serious body armor—muscle—and then maintain it while they systematically develop enough endurance to go the distance. That balance between muscularity and conditioning is a delicate one to achieve, and never more so than when he takes a client like me out on the road. If I catch a cold on tour and cancel a date, a lot of money is at stake for many people, including the promoter, let alone thousands of disappointed fans. Scooter knows exactly how far he can push me, just as he knows exactly how far we can push you in the Platinum Workout.

I may look like a pro athlete, but at the end of the day, I'm an artist and a businessman. I'm not looking to enter a World's Strongest Man contest. I'm looking to build an aesthetic body that can blow people away onstage, on-screen, or in a video. I don't have to prove how strong I am; I need to present a certain look. And when I'm performing, I need to be in good enough cardiovascular shape to move like an uncaged lion and sing at the same time.

Scooter: "After a while, you can read your client not only motivationally, to see if burnout is approaching, but also by monitoring his strength levels and his heart rate to see if he's overtraining. If LL was overtraining, he would tell me, 'Scooter, I'm beat. It's over. It's a wrap. Go relax.' Occasionally there would be stretches where we wouldn't work out for 2 or 3 days because he would be very tired. It's just not productive to train in that state.

"The goal is to keep the client very strong, and I do that by balancing food, supplementation, and rest along with working out. It's a very hard process to figure out for each individual, and I can't predict what all of your unique characteristics are going to be in advance. If I could do that, I'd be a million-dollar baby. It's trial and error, but the Platinum Workout gives you the blueprint enabling you to make your own adjustments as needed. Everyone has his own limitations. Everyone has his own wants and desires. LL happens to desire reaching a mountain peak. Then, when he gets to the mountain peak, he wants to jump up into the sky. And once he hits the sky he's like, 'Where do we go from here?'"

***We've tried enough things enough times to know what works and what doesn't work.*** This is what I mean by trial and error. When Scooter was working ringside with one of his first big fighters, Oleg Maskaev, he asked him if he could wear a heart rate monitor. "Oleg, please, just give me one round," he said.

Oleg goes, "No, I can't, because it's gonna—"

Scooter says, "Oleg, just give me one round, and I will tell you why."

When you're training at an elevated heart rate, you don't push yourself as much as you really can. When you start to reach the state of discomfort, naturally you have a tendency to back off. So what Scooter did was measure Oleg's heart rate in the uncomfortable state of actually fighting in the ring, which turned out to be 185 beats per minute. After that, in training, Scooter knew he needed to work Oleg in a range from 10 percent below to 5 percent above that. That way he grew accustomed to feeling that stress on his heart and his body, that intense fatigue. So when that fatigue hits you, you're used to it. You don't get nervous thinking, *Oh, I'm running out of gas—what am I going to do?* No. Whether it was Round 1 or Round 12 or Round 15, Scooter's fighters were always as fresh as possible because they had already fought the fight at the gym.

Here's how that approach translates to my world.

Scooter: "The hardest part of becoming a champion isn't the fight itself, it's training for that fight. And that's how Todd looks at everything. He looks forward to perfecting himself and his craft, his mind, his spirit—bringing it

Don't u call this a regular jam
I'm gonna rock this land
I'm gonna take this itty bitty world by storm
And I'm just gettin' warm
Just like Muhammad Ali they called him Cassius
Watch me bash this beat like a skull

—LL Cool J, **"Mama Said Knock You Out,"** 1990

all together to where he can stand onstage confident that he looks good, that he feels good, and that he's not going to get winded. So many of these singers now are putting tapes behind them. You saw Ashlee Simpson on *Saturday Night Live.* They use prerecorded tape, most of them. Todd is one of the originators. He doesn't use a tape. He's live. When you see 'live and in concert,' he's live and in concert. He's not live and on tape."

## Full Force

In the end, the results spoke for themselves. I learned a lot about conquering discomfort; I learned a lot about conquering that inner resistance that comes before you embark on any great undertaking; I learned that if I stick to it, I can make things happen, God willing. I found out that if you *really* want to do something, anything is possible. You can chop down a thousand trees in a row if you really want to. It's just a matter of getting up every day and goin' to work.

Yeah, that was the real deal. All told, the tour lasted about 3 months. I'm probably the first entertainer in history to pack on 12 pounds of muscle on the road while burning a bunch of body fat in the process. As for Scooter Pie? He went nuts. I found out he was crazy. In a good way. He lost 12 pounds trying to keep up with all of our craziness that goes from being on tour with a rap star. That's what you call a win-win situation.

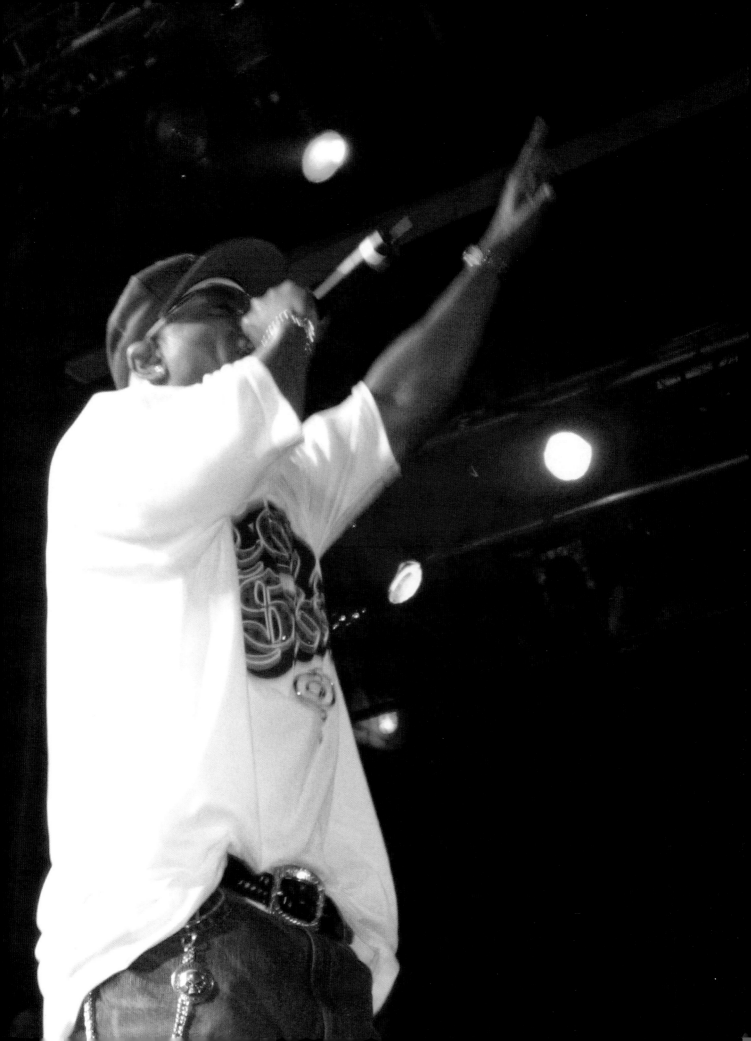

**Benefits achievable over 5 weeks:**

# 2 INCHES OFF YOUR WAIST

for those seeking significant body-fat reduction

# MUSCLES that appear MORE TONED

# 20 percent increase in ENERGY LEVELS

Measurable reductions in **BLOOD PRESSURE** and **BAD CHOLESTEROL**

hase one

# THE BRONZE BODY

## chapter two
# CHARGING THE PLATINUM BODY

**Action conquers fear.**
—PETER N. ZARLENGA

**D**URING WEEK 1 of the Platinum Workout, you're not going to work out. Before you lift a single weight, I want you to devote a week to doing nothing but putting your nutritional house in order. Heading straight to the gym is like launching a ship without sufficient fuel; you'll be adrift soon enough. Think of this week as "charging" up the platinum body.

Before you even break your first sweat, I'm going to take you through your kitchen for an extreme makeover, LL Cool J style. We're going to see what you've got in your food cabinets and fridge right now, tossing what you don't need in this big green can and adding things you do need to be successful with your new lifestyle. Ready? Let's rock!

First of all, the fridge. Let me tell you straight

up, I just opened it and it does not smell pretty. Here's what you've got:

Ooh! Is that bacon I see lying on a plate congealed in grease? That has got to go.

On the shelves, I see a package of 97% fat-free ground beef, eggs, a to-go container with congealed pasta Alfredo, some wheat bread, American cheese slices, and another container with…what is *that*? Chinese-Italian-Indian-Mexican-soul food, I think? It's so nasty, it could be anything.

In the produce drawer—which is filthy, by the way—is a bunch of wilted lettuce, some dried-up carrots, and…what is that? Corn? You say it's been in there for a month? Looks like a blue washcloth.

On the door you've got whole milk, OJ, butter,

ketchup, mustard, relish, pickles, beer, ranch dressing, teriyaki sauce, barbecue sauce, mayonnaise, crunchy peanut butter, and grape jelly.

In the freezer, I see French vanilla ice cream, a frozen four-cheese pizza, Popsicles, chicken wings, and a bag of frozen strawberries. What's that for? *Daiquiris?* Man, you need more help than I thought.

Okay, now the food cabinet.

There's Quaker strawberries-and-cream-flavored instant oatmeal, Oreos, Cheez-Its, microwave popcorn, and a bag of potatoes that are growing leaves down there—you see that? We've got a can of clam chowder, a couple of boxes of sugary cereals, a jar of instant coffee, and bacon bits.

There's also a liter jug of Coke, a liter jug of root beer, and another liter jug of Sprite.

We've got corn oil, salt, and pepper.

In the back are some old potato chips, a box of white instant rice, and a can of black beans. What's this—Oscar Mayer Lunchables cheese and crackers? You in the third grade or something?

Man, you need help!

First, let's tackle the fridge. The number one thing to do straight off is to clean that monster— there's some serious bacteria growing in here! Use some hot water with a bit of bleach or soap, and wash it inside from top to bottom, especially the veggie drawer. And buy a couple boxes of baking soda to absorb the odor in there. No lie, it smells like feet!

Now it's time to restock. You've got some good stuff going on with your 97% fat-free ground beef,

whole-wheat bread, eggs, OJ, and the attempt at having some veggies. But the rest of it has either got to go completely or be modified to better fit your new Platinum workouts. Here are my suggestions.

Swap your American cheese slices for fat-free or low-fat cheese, and trade your whole milk for fat-free or 1% milk.

Instead of regular butter, try Smart Balance spread or I Can't Believe It's Not Butter spray.

Your condiments look all right, but I would suggest fat-free or low-fat mayo and fat-free ranch dressing instead of the regular kind. And always remember to use things like teriyaki and barbecue sauce sparingly to avoid loading up on salt and extra calories.

Personally, I'd trade the commercial peanut butter for an all-natural one, such as Laura Scudders or something freshly ground from a natural-foods store. Processed peanut butter contains added sugar, oil, and salt, whereas all-natural ones contain only one ingredient: peanuts. The same goes for the jelly. I'd recommend a real fruit jelly or jam instead of one with added sugar.

As for the to-go containers, if you don't eat your leftovers the very next day, throw them out. Food that sits like that is a breeding ground for bacteria, and nasty stuff like that that can give new meaning to the old-school hip-hop term *illin'.*

The same goes for that bacon sitting there. You've got to put food in a container or zipper-lock bag to keep it fresh and bacteria free. And speaking of bacon, as good as that stuff tastes, kick it to

**LL 'S FAT-BURNING TIP** Think of the grocery store as a track, and do 90 percent of your shopping in the running lanes on the outside; stay off the infield. This will limit your intake of unhealthy fats (especially trans fats) and calories. The stores are nearly all set up the same way: produce on one side, meats and fish in the back, and dairy and bread on the other side. All the stuff you shouldn't be eating is in the middle.

the curb. Try some turkey bacon instead. It has a much lower fat content than pork bacon.

If you need to indulge in or entertain with alcohol, have some light beer handy instead of the regular stuff. And for God's sake, get something better than Old Mil! That's just embarrassing.

Fresh vegetables are in seriously short supply here. A good way to make sure you eat them before they disintegrate is to slice them into snackable portions as soon as you arrive home from the store, and then put them into clear containers in plain view on the shelves. And if you're into salad, bagged salad greens, spinach, and collard greens stay fresh longer than the loose stuff. If you just can't get it together with the fresh veggies, get some frozen ones instead. They keep longer and cook up in a flash in the microwave.

Speaking of the freezer, eighty-six that ice cream. One pint is so full of fat and calories, you would have to skip a whole day's meals to make up for it! Instead of the sugary Popsicles, I recommend the Real Fruit Bars, which are made with fruit juice and chunks of fruit instead.

Swap those chicken wings, which have very little meat on them, for chicken breasts, pork chops, lean steaks, fish fillets, and ground turkey.

# GETTING STARTED: YOUR WEEK 1 CHECKLIST

Here's a breakdown of all the things you should do to prep yourself for the training portion of the Platinum Workout, which begins in Week 2. Notice that some of this information is a little repetitive. That's the point—the success of my program is all in the reps. Once you grow accustomed to eating six meals and drinking eight glasses of water each and every day, it becomes second nature. By spending a week enforcing the pattern of good habits, you'll be that much ahead of the game when you start your workouts.

## Monday

• Clean out your refrigerator as outlined in this chapter.

• Get rid of old condiments (the ones with dry crust on the rim).

• Make a grocery list, including:

  • Condiments that you've just thrown out

  • Spices (cinnamon, cayenne pepper, basil, etc.)

  • Lean meats

  • Lean fish (such as tuna) and fatty fish (such as salmon)

  • Plenty of fruit and vegetables

  • Healthy foods that enhance flavor (lemons, lime, garlic, ginger)

• Go grocery shopping.

• Buy a workout journal.

• Make a simple dinner: lean grilled steak and vegetables.

## Tuesday

• Clean out your cupboards (get rid of all the junk food that's likely to tempt you).

• Make a few multiple-ingredient foods such as chicken vegetable soup, turkey chili, etc., to have on hand when you don't have time to cook.

• Freeze individual servings of these healthy foods.

• Eat at least five small meals throughout the day.

• Record the meals in your workout journal.

## Wednesday

• Eat at least five small meals throughout the day.

As for the frozen cheese pizza, well, you know what to do with that! You can actually make your own healthy pizza out of one of those Boboli crusts, some sauce, a few spices, lots of veggies, grilled chicken, and a little bit of fat-free mozzarella.

Now, on to the food cabinet. First of all, here's a tip: When plants start to grow, that food is no longer edible. Either throw out those old potatoes or plant them in the backyard and grow your own crop. Either way, get 'em outta there without a moment's hesitation. And again, give everything a good cleaning with bleach and water before restocking. You're kind of messy.

Okay, here we go:

While we're on the subject of potatoes, in addition to the regular baking kind, I'd add a few yams and sweet potatoes to your stock. They digest more slowly and stick with you longer as well as having tons of vitamins and minerals.

Your instant oatmeal cereal is a better breakfast choice than sweetened cereal, but I recommend making plain oatmeal and flavoring it with fresh fruit and low-fat milk instead. The instant packets have a lot of preservatives and processed sugar that you don't need going into your body.

- Download workout music to your iPod in preparation for the workouts to come.

- Drink eight glasses of water.

- Take your multivitamin.

- Record the meals in your workout journal.

### Thursday

- Join a gym or get your home gym equipment ready to go.

- Eat six small meals throughout the day.

- Drink eight glasses of water.

- Take your multivitamin.

- Record the meals in your workout journal.

### Friday

- Eat six small meals throughout the day.

- Drink eight glasses of water.

- Take your multivitamin.

- Buy gym clothes and shoes to help get you motivated for your workouts.

- Record the meals in your workout journal.

### Saturday

- Eat six small meals throughout the day.

- Drink eight glasses of water.

- Take your multivitamin.

- Enjoy a reward such as a cookie or glass of wine if you've successfully followed your meal plan throughout the week.

- Record the meals in your workout journal.

### Sunday

- Eat six small meals throughout the day.

- Drink eight glasses of water.

- Take your multivitamin.

- Hit the grocery store and restock. Emphasize a range of foods, but also buy plenty of the ones you know you're going to eat frequently (eggs, egg whites, chicken breasts, broccoli, etc.).

- Record the meals in your workout journal.

All those cookies, snack foods, and cakes have got to go, as do the sugary cereals and bacon bits. Do you even know what's in a bacon bit? All I know is it sure ain't bacon. Read the ingredients. (As a rule of thumb, if a product contains more than 20 ingredients and the label reads like a chemistry experiment, throw it out.) Replace those unhealthy snack foods with whole-wheat crackers, dried fruit, raw nuts, trail mix, even whole-wheat pretzels.

The microwave popcorn is a good idea, but buy the light or reduced-sodium versions instead of the regular ones. Better yet, buy yourself an air-popper or microwave popping bowl (they sell them at Wal-Mart), pop it up, then put on some I Can't Believe It's Not Butter spray, some salt substitute, even some Splenda for kettle-corn style.

All that regular soda is superhigh in sugar and needs to be tossed out and replaced with either diet soda, regular water, or sparkling water. Coffee is fine, but I would also add some decaf green tea for antioxidants.

Soup can be a good meal, but instead of clam chowder, which is cream based and chock-full of calories and fat, buy lighter, healthier options such

# 9 WAYS TO BURN 100 CALORIES

The Platinum Workout is a hard-core program designed to get you in the shape of your life. But little, easy-to-do things can help make it easier for you to reach your goal. Consider incorporating some of these minor lifestyle adjustments into your daily routine to complement your regular training.

**1. Take the stairs.** If you consistently use elevators or escalators to move from one level to the next, you can take advantage of your tiered lifestyle to help you shape up. Using the stairs can help increase the amount of calories you burn on a daily basis. Feel free to go up and down a few extra times, too. You may be surprised by how challenging walking stairs can become after only a minute or two. After all, most of us are only used to walking up one flight of stairs here or there.

**2. Eat six meals every day.** I stress this throughout the Platinum Workout: If you eat six meals a day, you'll be surprised that you're never hungry *and* that you're shedding body fat. Every time you eat, it causes your body to burn calories—digestion is a highly active physiological process. So, if you're eating 2,000 calories a day, you'll burn many more calories if you divide them equally into six meals than you will if you divide them into three. In other

words, digesting twice as much food at one meal doesn't take twice as many calories. Initiating the process of digestion is where you get the calorie-burning advantage.

**3. Cut the portions.** While this holds true no matter how many meals a day you eat, it's particularly true if you're eating six times a day. Portion management is as crucial as the number of meals you're eating every day. Cut back so that most of your meals are only 300 to 400 calories apiece. This sometimes means that your meals will consist of two foods at a time. Examples of balanced smaller meals include a bagel with cream cheese, a small portion (4 ounces) of chicken breast with a generous serving of a steamed vegetable, or a moderate-size bowl of vegetable beef soup.

**4. Cut back on dessert.** Can you eat dessert on this program? Yes. Should you eat a large amount of cake or a handful of cookies? No. Should you eat dessert every day? No. Portion management and frequency are two of the best ways to control calories. If you're regularly eating dessert, cut it out most days of the week. But don't cut it out altogether. Once or twice a week, allow yourself a small treat, and think of this as a reward instead of falling off the wagon. (The idea that you've fallen off the wagon can lead to overindulging with that "I've already blown my diet, so there's nothing I can do; I might as well keep eating" attitude. Avoid this type of thinking.)

There's no forgettin' this, the way I'm reppin' this
My bodyguard's big but do that
## make me weaponless
I'm in the Hamptons,
# game stronger than Sampson
That's why I'm still a teen pop idol like Hanson

—LL Cool J, **"I'm About To Get Her," 2004**

---

**5. Exercise when you watch TV.** Most people find time to watch at least an hour of TV a day. For others, that's just their warmup. If you take time to turn on the tube, you can also exercise while you watch it. Consider acquiring a piece of cardio equipment that you can use while viewing, or take this time to perform your daily stretch. If this is more than you can handle, another way to increase your metabolic rate is to find nonexercise activities (such as cleaning or straightening up) to perform while you watch TV. Even simply standing burns significantly more calories than lounging on the couch.

**6. Get a good stretch first thing in the morning.** Stretching is crucial to your overall training program. By maintaining or improving your flexibility, you will not only help to prevent injury but you'll also encourage better muscular development through better posture and muscle control. You can do this right when you wake up to get your blood flowing. Not only will you feel better but your metabolism will get a jump start as you begin burning calories from the start of the day.

**7. Drink black coffee.** Like I say throughout the book, I'm not a big believer in fat burners as a miracle cure to give you the body you want. Still, energy management is a tool to help you achieve what you want for your body. Drinking black coffee serves a few different functions. First, coffee jacks up your metabolic rate, helping you burn more calories each day. Second, black coffee contains virtually no calories, so you're not adding to fat stores when you drink it. (This is especially true if you were previously adding cream and sugar to your coffee.) Third, coffee can actually inhibit your appetite so you want to consume fewer calories.

**8. Go for a walk at lunch.** If you work a traditional 9-to-5, you probably spend much of your day sitting in a chair behind a desk. But almost everyone gets a lunch hour, and you should take advantage of yours to burn some calories. A 20- or 30-minute walk at lunch every day (even if you're just going someplace to get your lunch) can really add up. Not only that, you'll have more energy in the afternoon, particularly if you accelerate the pace of the walk a bit.

**9. Superset or shorten the rest period between weight sets.** A nice long rest between weight-training sets allows your body to recover to full strength so it can perform more reps in the next set. While this strategy can maximize muscle building, it isn't necessarily the most efficient way to burn calories. When you shorten the rest period to about 30 to 45 seconds between sets, you'll jack up the cardiovascular requirements placed upon your body, and you'll burn significantly more calories during an hour-long workout, even if you need to drop weights or reps.

# S COOTER'S *MUSCLE-BUILDING TIP*

Skip the caffeine after dinner. A review published in the journal *Sleep* noted that 70 percent of a male's growth hormone is released shortly after the onset of sleep, so you're probably sacrificing muscle growth if you're still tossing and turning past midnight. And caffeine typically lingers in your system for 4 to 6 hours.

as vegetable barley or chicken and rice. Also, carefully check the sodium content of the cans. Buy a ready-made low-sodium soup.

Rice and beans make a great meal because when eaten together, they contain the full spectrum of amino acids. But I would definitely replace the white instant rice with whole-grain or wild rice. If you're time crunched, the quick stuff is okay, but it's heavily processed and won't stick with you long. Also, beware of the sodium content of the canned beans. Buy brands that are lower in sodium, and rinse them well before eating to wash away excess salt and preservatives.

Replace your corn oil with extra-virgin olive oil, and expand your seasoning horizons to include more than salt and pepper. Try some of the Mrs. Dash blends, an assortment of dried herbs and spices, or salt-free seasonings on meats, poultry, and fish.

Instead of prepackaged lunches made with some orange processed crap, make your own Platinum fat-free-cheese-and-whole-wheat-cracker lunch to take to work.

Finally, I would add a can of whey protein powder to your cabinet—whatever flavor you like. A smoothie or shake is a great meal on the go, and you could put those frozen strawberries to better use than in daiquiris.

So there you go. We've purged your kitchen of any food sabotage possible, and we've suggested tons of new foods and ideas to improve your nutrition here at home. I know you'll stick to your new eating plan for sure and get the platinum body you've always wanted.

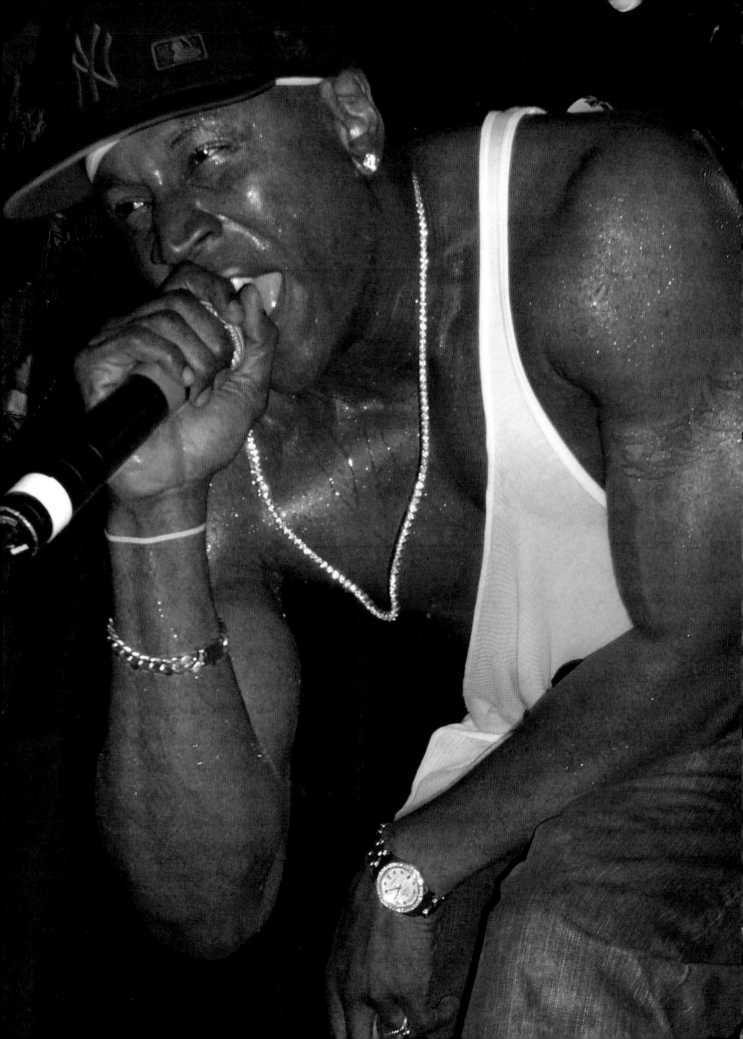

# chapter three
# IT'S TIME TO WORK OUT

**The time is always right to do what is right.**
—MARTIN LUTHER KING JR.

**D**URING THIS first month of actual training, which coincides with Weeks 2 through 5 of the program—remember, Week 1 was devoted to getting your kitchen in order and getting ready to train—you'll start down the road to the best shape of your life. Full-body training done three times a week will expose muscle fibers to resistance, and several aerobic sessions will get your cardiorespiratory system pumping like it should be.

So let's get right into this, shall we?

The first thing you're going to notice is that we start you off using machines exclusively. You might wonder about this, as you're probably used to working out with free weights. If you think machines aren't for people serious about getting a hard

body, think again. There's nothing inherently wrong with machines where muscle growth is concerned. You can overload a muscle just as well with a machine as you can with a free weight. I know at least one pro bodybuilder who says that if he wants to overload a muscle and recruit it for growth and strength, he uses machines.

The main difference with machines is that you're lifting in a fixed plane. Ultimately, that becomes a limitation. Here's why: In a fixed plane, you don't have to worry about balance or stability, so all those little helper muscles that normally come into play with free weights can basically stand on the sidelines and twiddle their thumbs. That's a double-edged sword, though, because if you were using free weights early on, those helper muscles could also fatigue and then fail before you had maxed out the effects on the bigger target muscles.

That's one gold star for machines, but their advantage comes at the very beginning of a program. The reason we're having you start with, say, a machine bench press instead of a bench press with free weights is ease of use. As a beginner, you probably don't have a training partner, a personal trainer, or certainly as much knowledge as you will have when you finish this book. When you pick up a set of dumbbells, rest assured you won't find any instructions written on them. Instead, we're going to ask you to use a machine that has the guidelines plastered on the side in plain English. "Sit here," "adjust the seat pad," "grab this handle"—I'm talking see-Spot-run kind of stuff here. You can easily get in or on the machine, safely execute the exercise, and develop a feel for the groove of that particular movement. Combining machine moves early, as we've done in the Platinum Workout, is really the best introduction to resistance training.

For the sake of argument, let's pretend that you've gotten past that initial point of knowing how to perform certain free-weight exercises, even a bunch of them. We *still* want you to start with machines. For these 2 or 3 weeks, you're going to be dealing with a lot of what's called delayed-onset muscle soreness (meaning it sets in a day or two after the actual workout) and other things you've never experienced before. As of yet, you haven't developed the neurological adaptations needed for free weights.

Say what—neurological adaptations? Isn't this about lifting weights to make your muscles grow? Ultimately, yes, but initially your body is more concerned with learning how to do exercises than with sprouting Popeye muscle. And "learning" in this case is mainly a function of your body's nervous system. It's so much easier for a beginner to learn to control the eccentric contraction—usually the lowering of the weight—on a machine than with a dumbbell, for instance. At this stage of the game, we don't necessarily want you to worry about all of the different facets that free weights bring into play. We don't want you worrying about balance. We don't want you obsessing over safety. We want you to learn the movements themselves, like going through an explosive upstroke followed by a controlled return down.

Safety also argues for starting on machines. To some extent, well-made machines are pretty much dummy-proof. The apparatus automatically places you in a position of biomechanical advantage for that particular move, meaning they make your body move how it's supposed to. In contrast, for a bench press with dumbbells, you've got to pick up the weights, sit down with them, and position them in the correct starting position. Only then can you begin pressing. In contrast, you sit in or on a machine according to the instructions and then start lifting. If you choose the wrong weight with a machine, you can just let the handles back down, pull out the pin, and place it in a lighter (or heavier, if it's too easy) slot. In contrast, if you're pressing dumbbells and find yourself in a really awkward, uncomfortable situation, you're suddenly at risk of injury as you attempt a "safe landing."

**LL'S FAT-BURNING TIP** Find a meaningful reason and challenge yourself to give up a food addiction, such as sweets for Christmas. After a few weeks of doing without, you may not even want it anymore.

Last but not least, we're having you use machines for the first 2 weeks because researchers have determined that they are more effective at initiating the process of muscle growth in greenhorns. This ties in with the fact that machine moves are easier for your central nervous system to master initially.[1]

In the long term, compound exercises such as the squat and deadlift, which allow you to move more weight, can't be beat for building muscle. I swear by them. And by the time we ask you to perform those moves, you already will have developed the strength, flexibility, and neuromuscular coordination needed to master them. But at the start, the learning curve is a little steeper—and your body won't really start gaining muscle until that curve has been overcome.

## Wired Tight with Circuits

We're also going to start you off with a workout style called circuit training, which refers to doing exercises consecutively, with little or no rest separating them. I love circuit training because it allows me to accomplish a lot of work done in a little bit of time. Then I can be off to do my next thing. A great workout for me is 45 minutes where I get it on and poppin', and then hit the exit pumped like a basketball. Also, studies have shown repeatedly that this training style increases lean mass and aerobic capacity while reducing body fat.

Depending on how the circuit is designed, it can range from something comfortably undertaken by beginners (how we've done it for these first few weeks) to something incredibly hard (you'll experience that later on in the Platinum Workout).

In large part, because circuit training is so efficient, actors like me have used it to shape up for film roles for decades. To illustrate just how hard circuit training can be, I'd like to share a short anecdote about one of my early film heroes, Sylvester Stallone. Even to an African-American kid born and raised in Queens, Sly embodied machismo through his portrayals of muscular antiheroes such as down-and-out prizefighter Rocky Balboa and disillusioned Vietnam vet John Rambo. (Mr. T in *Rocky III* was especially inspirational for me. He was like, "I got a prediction for the fight: Pain!" Yo, that was the best *Rocky* out of all of them! *Rocky III* was *hot*! I'm tellin' ya.) Anyway, excuse the digression—the point is that guns resembling pythons soon became standard issue for action-adventure stars and inspiration for aspiring actors like me.

You would just assume, then, that Sly only trained the old-fashioned way, pushing iron around the gym like bodybuilders and powerlifters. Well, not long after the first *Rocky* was released, Sly was training at a Bally's gym in Hollywood; there, too, as part of his roving responsibilities as director of education for the gym chain was the legendary strength coach Dr. Paul Ward, a former Marine who had gone on to play offensive

---

[1] *Here's how we know this. Researchers from McMaster University in Hamilton, Ontario, Canada, divided 29 women into two groups (Chilibeck P., Calder A., Sale D., Webber C. "A comparison of strength and muscle mass increase during resistance training in young women." European Journal of Applied Physiology. 77:170–175, 1998). Nineteen of them worked out doing bench presses, leg curls, and biceps curls, along with several other moves, for 20 weeks. Ten of them didn't exercise. The workout group was further divided into two groups: 10 who did all the exercises on 1 day twice a week, and 9 who followed an upper-body/lower-body split routine.*

*While everyone who trained gained strength and built muscle over the 20 weeks, muscle gains were most dramatic during the first 10 weeks on the barbell curl, a single-joint move—as are most machines. Similarly, other studies have concluded that single-joint exercises produce muscle gains the fastest, while multijoint moves produce muscle gains initially—and that is a huge qualifier here—at a slower pace.*

*By the way, if you guys out there are dismissing this research as irrelevant to you because the subjects were female, realize that other studies have shown that men and women adapt to resistance training the same way during the first 4 months of training.*

line for the Detroit Lions. Since leaving the NFL, he had conducted several of the groundbreaking studies proving the effectiveness of a new exercise concept called—you guessed it—circuit training.

Dr. Ward recalls: "I didn't recognize him because I hadn't seen the movie yet, but the area supervisor for Bally's said, 'Hey, that's the guy in *Rocky*—you want to meet him?' I said, 'Yeah, sure,' so we walked over there, and Sylvester started telling me how hard he had trained for his movie. I said, 'Have you ever tried circuit weight training?'

"He said, 'No. What is it?'

"I told him about doing 10 or so exercises more or less nonstop, going from one station to the next and alternating muscle groups, all while getting your heart rate up to between 130 and 160 beats per minute. What makes it unique, I continued, is that it taxes your aerobic and anaerobic energy systems and everything in between simultaneously.

"He said, 'Sounds good! Let's try it.'"

With everyone in the gym gathered round, Sly blasted through three circuits, only to disappear immediately afterward. "So I wander out onto the sunroof track, and there's Sylvester, lying back in a chair with one foot propped up on a table, totally exhausted," recalls Ward, who was both shocked and impressed that an actor could run such a gauntlet. "Eventually, he heads toward the john, and I'm thinking, *I'll wait till he gets out to congratulate him.* But when he came out, the guy was *totally* wiped out."

For you young heads reading this, *Rambo* is a cool movie. Make sure you rent a copy. And then get a massage.

At the beginning of the Platinum Workout, your circuits will be far, far kinder and gentler than the ones that made Rocky pray to the porcelain goddess. But later in the Platinum Workout, once your body has been prepped to handle it, Scoots will throw some circuits your way that definitely will challenge your inner Rambo.

## THE PLATINUM BURGER

Burgers can be great for you—they offer a load of important vitamins and minerals, such as zinc and iron, along with a hefty dose of protein. Unfortunately, they can also pack in a lot of calories and fat, much of it saturated. However, there's a way to make them better for you and limit the downside. Here's how.

Start with the following ingredients:

4 ounces lean red meat

Pepper (applied to taste)

¼ cup chopped red onion

Lettuce and tomato

1 whole-wheat hamburger bun

Once you've assembled the building materials, do the following:

**1.** Heat the grill.

**2.** Place an ice cube on the grill grates. (Whatever you do, don't fry the burger.)

**3.** When it melts, the grill is hot and ready for you to cook.

**4.** Mix the red meat, pepper, and onion, forming the ingredients into a patty that looks like a hockey puck.

**5.** Place the burger on the heated grill and cook for approximately 4 minutes on each side, or until the juices are no longer red.

**6.** Once cooked, top the burger with lettuce and tomato. Leave off the bacon.

**7.** Put the burger, which should be the size of a deck of cards, on a whole-wheat bun and top with ketchup, mustard, or salsa. Skip the mayo.

*Totals: 412 calories, 44 grams of carbohydrates, 31 grams of protein, 11 grams of fat*

—Christopher R. Mohr, PhD, RD

## SLEIGHT-OF-HAND CAN MEAN BIG RESULTS

"Get a grip." "Can you handle it?" "Dropping the ball." If you don't think hand positioning is important—get your mind out of the gutter—rummage through America's pop-culture expressions and see how many of the most commonly used ones reference the hold we have on things. See, there's another.

Never is this more true than when you hit the gym. Inside, you'll see an array of equipment designed to work the body in a dizzying variety of ways. Barbells, dumbbells, machines, cable setups...they're all different, but for nearly all of them to work, you're going to have to place your hand on *something* first, even if it's just to support your body while you train legs.

How you grip those apparatus matters. A lot. On the one hand, you can use two hands to assume a grip as wide as possible, whether that means sliding your hands to the far ends of an Olympic bar, or grasping the D handles of a cable stack for crossovers. (You'll learn what D handles are in a second.) Alternatively, you could place both hands right next to each other, so that your fingers are actually touching. Most grips fall somewhere between these two extremes.

Here are the main reasons why grip is so important. First, when you're training big, strong muscles like your chest and back, you don't want your forearms and wrists to give way before the muscles

themselves do, because then you're not getting a complete workout. Second, the fibers in your muscles fire differently for a given exercise depending on what your grip is, and change is good for muscles, as we emphasize throughout *Platinum Workout*. (On upright rows, for example, a wide grip hits more deltoids, less traps. A narrow grip hits less traps, more deltoids.) Third, holding a heavy weight the wrong way can injure your wrists faster than you say "ouch"! Fourth, and last, who doesn't want an iron grip? Our handshake is often the first thing people notice about us.

As a general rule, when you're using both arms at once on a cable exercise for your back, you'll be using some sort of bar handle. It might be long or short, straight or curved, chrome or steel; regardless, it will enable you to pull on a weight stack using your lat muscles. When you're training triceps or biceps, bars again will come in handy (rope handles also work well for triceps). For shoulders, D-type handles, a.k.a. stirrup handles, often will be your first choice for exercises such as the cable lateral raise. These smaller handles are great for training one arm at a time.

*Suffice it to say that when Scooter and I recommend using a particular handle on a certain exercise, we do so for good reason. Nothing is arbitrary or random in the Platinum Workout.* So make every effort to find and use that particular handle, bearing in mind that the world won't end if you can't—use something else instead. Doing the exercise with *something* is at least 90 percent of the battle.

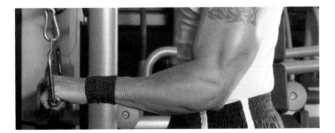

**1. Overhand grip:** When you reach up for something such as a bar dangling from a high cable pulley, this is how most people would instinctively grasp it: by placing their palm atop the bar and wrapping their fingers over and around it, except for their thumb, which goes underneath.

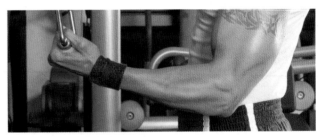

**2. Underhand grip:** In this scenario, you would grasp the bar or handle with your palms touching the bottom of it and your fingers wrapping up and over, except for your thumb or thumbs, which would wrap in the reverse direction. This is also sometimes referred to as a reverse grip because it's the opposite of the standard overhand grip. Sometimes we'll ask you to use this grip for cable pulls because it places the lats in a maximally stretched position prepull.

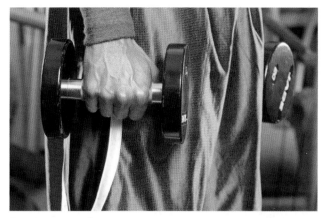

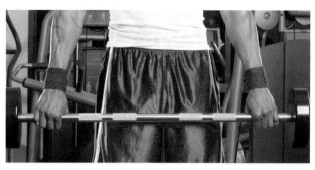

**6. Wide grip:** Regardless of your wrist orientation, overhand or underhand, this typically means your hands lie outside of your shoulders.

**3. Neutral grip:** Here your palms actually face each other. Some attachments have cylinders at either end of the bar with small bars running perpendicular to the main bar, allowing your palms to face each other. Alternatively, the bar might be bent into a V at the end, permitting the same wrist orientation through different means.

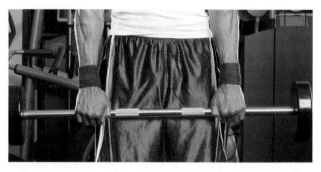

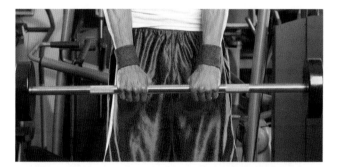

**7. Thumbless grip:** This means keeping your thumb on the same side of the grip as your other fingers, rather than wrapping it underneath. It's often used to lessen the influence of the biceps.

**4. Narrow grip:** Regardless of your wrist orientation, overhand or underhand, your hands are relatively close together in this situation.

Again, don't become hung up on learning the technicalities of this stuff (unless you want to, in which case, go for it). Learn enough to do what you need to do when you see a grip or hand placing mentioned in the book—and then let the results speak for themselves.

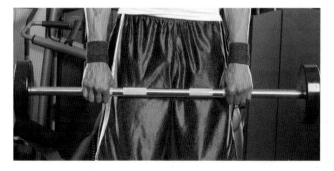

**5. Shoulder-width grip:** Regardless of your wrist orientation, overhand or underhand, your hands are aligned directly with your shoulders.

**LL'S STRENGTHEN-YOUR-GRIP TIP** Carry a tennis ball around with you and practice squeezing it when you're stuck in line or traffic.

# The Weighting Game

So how much weight should you lift? We want to make weight selection as easy as possible for you. Most programs ask you to determine your maximum lift for one repetition—which sometimes becomes apparent only when the bar or dumbbells come crashing into your rib cage. (Let's leave that one-rep maximum stuff for guys who pull tractors on ESPN, shall we?) Then they ask you to calculate a percentage of that weight, assuming you carry a calculator with you to the gym.

*In the Platinum Workout, through some quick trial and error, you simply find the weight that causes you to sacrifice correct form for the first time within the prescribed rep range.* (We're talking about the weight that breaks you down just as you reach the desired number of reps.) The rep ranges determine your weight; the ranges aren't determined by the weight. You'll be able to handle heavier weights as your rep ranges fall.

# Weeks 2 and 3: Circuit Training

- Warm up for 5 to 10 minutes using a treadmill, a stationary bike, or some other cardio apparatus before each workout. Jumping jacks or running in place will also do the trick.
- In Week 2, choose machines that allow you to perform the movement described under "Full-

## MAKE GOOD FORM YOUR NORM

*There are right ways and wrong ways to lift hunks of metal.* I can't stress this point strongly enough. If it's not the most important point in the book, it's up there. For the same reason weights are so good for you—they can tax your body's muscle fibers and skeletal structure in ways that make them stronger—they can do a lot of damage if lifted incorrectly. Remember the skeleton in science class that used to dance in the breeze every time someone opened the door? That's *you.* That's how fragile your body is. When you lift heavy objects in ways that subject it to unnatural force, very bad things can start to happen. "Ninety percent of the time that injuries occur in the weight room, it's from someone using incorrect technique," says Jeffrey M. McBride, PhD, CSCS, an associate professor of biomechanics in the department of health, leisure, and exercise science at Appalachian State University in Boone, North Carolina.

"Whenever you're doing any exercise such as a deadlift or a squat, it all comes down to how your hips are positioned," says Dr. McBride when asked about the most common form blunders of beginners. "Basically, you need to have a slight anterior pelvic tilt. That means your lower back is in a concave position, with your chest out, as opposed to having a flat or rounded back. That's the position from which your body is designed to exert force."

When that position becomes compromised, it's often because someone is using too much weight—and *that* has to do with ego. Weight training and pride like to bump heads a lot. Right out of the chute, guys want to be heaving around weights worthy of Arnold Schwarzenegger back in the day. For a while, your body can handle it. Eventually, it surrenders.

*Good form not only prevents injuries but also leads to better results.* Your muscles don't remember the number of pounds you lifted or whether they came in the form of gold-plated dumbbells or cinder blocks in the backyard. They only remember the amount of stress you subjected them to. And as your muscles grow in response to this stimulus, you'll find yourself handling heavier weights in due time. So it's a win-win situation.

In the end, the only person you need to impress in the gym is the man or woman in the mirror.

Body Circuit." **Follow the how-to instructions on the frame of each machine.** During Week 3, where possible, switch to different machines for the same body part and movement. For example, consider going from a low-rowing machine in Week 2 to a high-rowing one in Week 3 or from a flat-bench press machine to an incline one.

- If you don't have access to a gym and machines but have weights at home, use the free-weight alternatives given below each machine.

- Do 15 reps of every set.

- Doing each exercise in succession from start to finish completes one circuit. Do one complete circuit in Week 2 and then two circuits in Week 3.

- Rest 30 seconds between sets.

- After completing each machine workout in Week 2, walk on the treadmill at 55 percent of maximum heart rate for 10 minutes. (Your MHR is 220 minus your age. Multiply this number by 0.55 to arive at 55 percent of MHR.) During Week 3, increase the time to 15 minutes while staying at 55 percent.

- Do this workout three times a week, always separating weight-training days by at least 48 hours. So if your first session of the week occurs, say, Monday night, don't lift weights again until Wednesday night at the earliest.

## FULL-BODY CIRCUIT

### Quads
Leg-press or leg-extension machine
(Alternative: barbell squat)

### Back
Rowing machine
(Alternative: one-arm dumbbell row)

### Abs
Crunch machine
(Alternative: crunch)

### Chest
Pressing machine
(Alternative: dumbbell bench press)

### Triceps
Triceps machine
(Alternative: dumbbell kickback)

### Biceps
Biceps machine
(Alternative: standing barbell curl)

### Shoulders
Overhead-press machine
(Alternative: seated dumbbell press)

### Hamstrings
Lying or standing leg curl machine
(Alternative: exercise ball leg curl)

## SCOOTER'S *STAY-MOTIVATED TIP*
Keep your workout clothes beside your bed the night before an early-morning workout. That way, when the alarm goes off, you won't hesitate.

# chapter four

# BEND SO YOU DON'T BREAK

**S**TRETCHING IS as crucial to working out as rehearsing is to filming a scene. When you see a muscle-bound guy, you probably assume that he can't move as well as an average person. Well, you're half right. Muscle-bound people are among the most and least flexible people on the planet. It all depends on whether they stretched as part of their muscle-building program. Keep in mind that muscle is a highly pliable tissue, and, within the realm of human possibility, it will do pretty much what you tell it you want it to do.

For best results, stretch every day, before or after your workout or between sets. My favorite is between sets because it keeps you active, and it keeps you opened up so you can use your full range of motion for the weight-training exercises

*A wise man can see more from the bottom of a well than a fool can from a mountaintop.*
*—Unknown*

you're performing during that workout. Stretching during workouts tends to counterbalance the muscle group you're working. For instance, when training your chest, a great stretch is opening your arms, grasping a post or weight rack, and stretching your pecs before you perform your next set.

You can also stretch for 5 to 15 minutes first thing in the morning or before bedtime. Keep in mind that stretching is exercise, too. If you do a lengthy stretch session right before your workout, you may find that a weight-training session is more challenging because you've already taxed your muscles.

Here's a rundown on some of the various types of stretching you can include in your program.

1. **Static stretching:** This is the most common type of stretching that you see in the gym and among the safest and most effective. It's the stretch-and-hold version. You move into a stretch and maintain it for 5 to 10 seconds, "sinking" into it and allowing your body to open up. For best results, perform at least three reps of static stretches—you'll find that you go deeper with each successive stretch.

2. **Active stretching (movement stretching):** Halfway between static and ballistic stretching lies active stretching, where you move smoothly between one stretch and the next. You go through the same range of motion as you do for static stretching, but you don't hold the stretch. Many underuse this form of stretching, but it can help open tight muscles. You often see athletes perform this type of stretch right before performance. Think of sprinters bending over to open their hamstrings or pulling their feet up behind them to open their quads.

3. **Ballistic stretching:** This type of stretching is one of the most effective, as well as one of the likeliest to cause injury. By adding dynamic force to your movement, you are able to take your range of motion beyond your static stretch position, helping to increase flexibility. Gymnasts often use ballistic stretches. My advice is to attempt this type of stretching only under the guidance of a qualified trainer.

4. **Passive stretching:** You see this a lot at the gym—a trainer stretching out a client. Passive stretching is when you relax and allow someone else to stretch you out. I think this type of stretching is great at the end of the workout as a way to relax and get a quick jump on the recovery process.

5. **Yoga:** Yoga has become enormously popular, and it's not only a great stretch but also a good workout. You might be surprised by how challenging it can be, especially if you're a little tight. (It's even more beneficial for those who are tighter than most.) Yoga can be performed at home with a tape or in a studio or gym as part of a class. You can also mix and match some of your favorites poses or stretches to create your own personal stretching routine.

6. **Pilates:** Similar to but slightly different from yoga, Pilates emphasizes control in movement, teaching you how to use your full range of motion properly as you tone and elongate your body. Joseph Pilates originally designed his moves and programs for injured dancers. Over the past decade, it has ballooned into one of the most popular fitness trends.

Here's a quick stretching routine that hits virtually the entire body using a combination of the techniques outlined above.

## SCOOTER'S *FAT-LOSS TIP*
Burn fat with protein. Researchers at McMaster University analyzed the diets of more than 600 individuals and found that those who ate 20 grams more protein than the group average collectively had a lower hips-to-waist ratio by 6 percent.

# Hamstrings (passive)
Lie flat on your back and lift one leg skyward. Have your training partner gently move that straight leg in the direction of your chest, and hold for several seconds. Repeat seven or eight times. Do the same number of reps using the other leg.

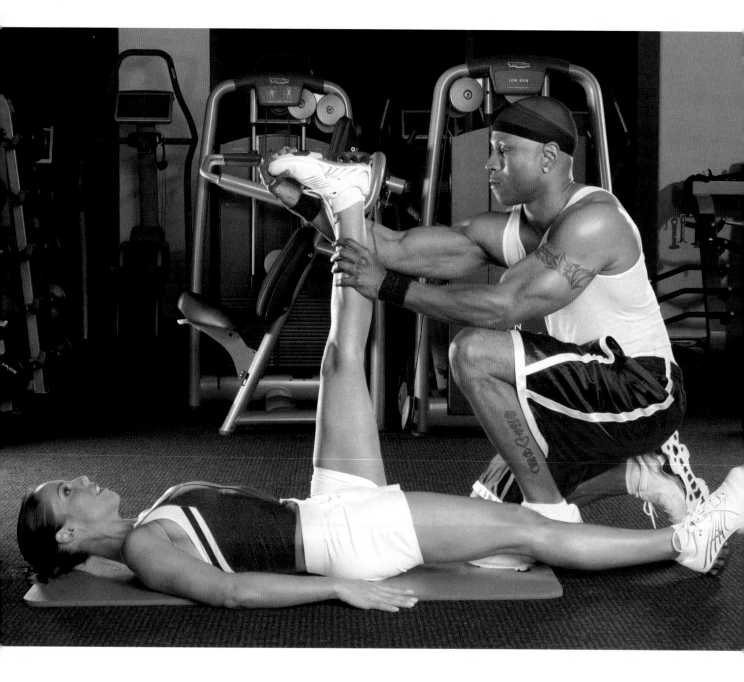

28

# Waist (active)
Stand up straight with your feet planted shoulder-width apart. Twist your torso to the right and then to the left. (That equals one stretch.) Repeat 20 to 25 times.

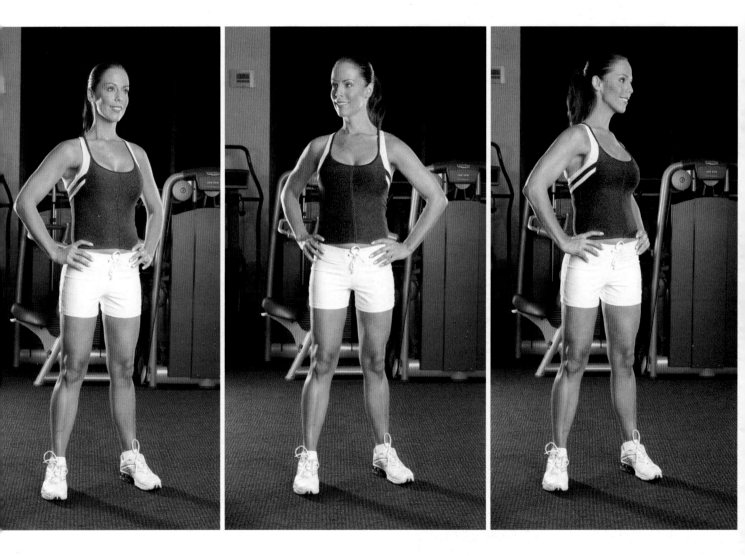

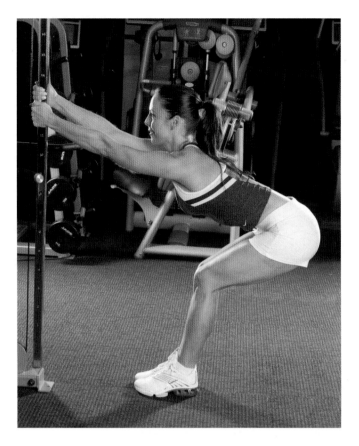

## Upper Back (static) Stand several feet away from a support you can grasp with both hands after leaning forward at the waist. Arch your back and hold that position for 10 to 20 seconds to stretch the upper half of your back.

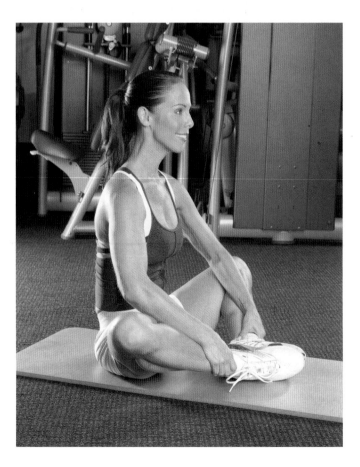

## Groin (static) Sit with your knees bent, so the soles of your feet are flush with each other. Use your elbows to press down gently on your knees until you feel a stretch spreading through your groin. Hold for 10 to 20 seconds. Repeat five times, pressing your knees down a little farther each time, if possible.

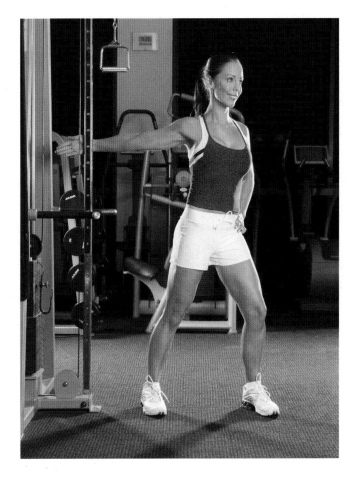

**Chest (static)** Stand next to a support and raise one arm until it's parallel to the floor and in the same plane as your shoulders. Shift one foot in front of the other and lean forward until you feel a nice stretch spreading across your chest. Hold this position for about 30 seconds, and then repeat using your other arm.

Daddy just made a nine-digit deposit
Believe me, sweetie, **it's not luck it's logic**
I'm the captain of my destiny
Used to dream of the things **I was blessed to see**

—LL Cool J, **"Amazin'," 2002**

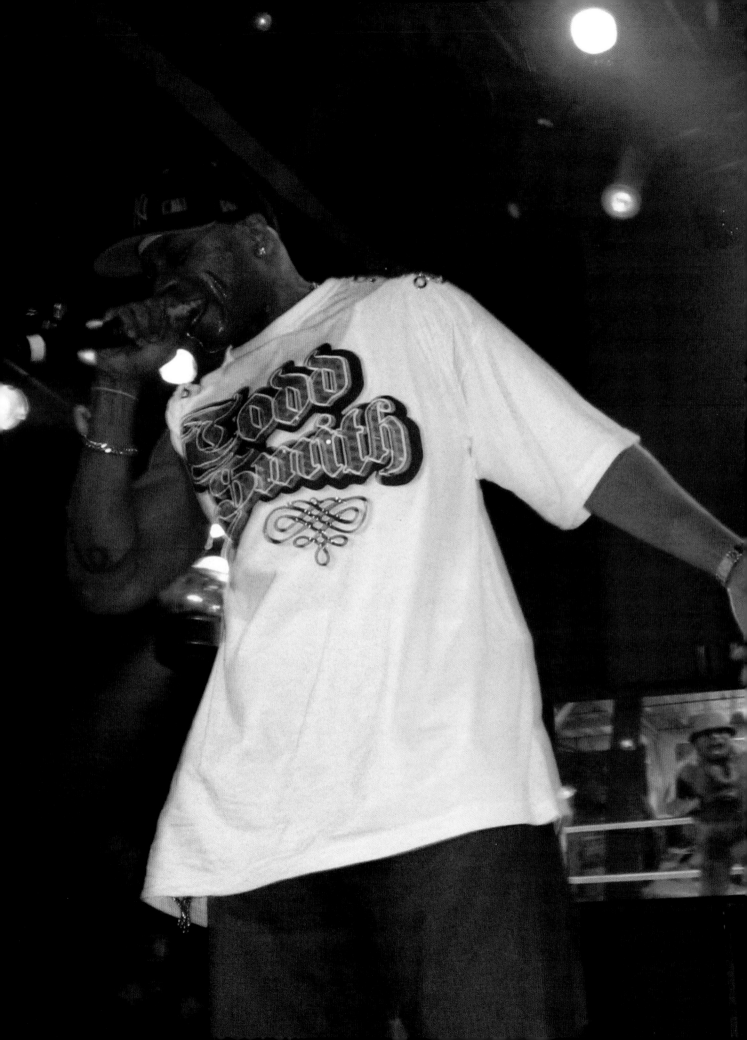

# chapter five

# GO PLATINUM WITH YOUR NUTRITION

**A** FITNESS-INDUSTRY rule of thumb states that nutrition is 80 percent of the equation when it comes to shaping up. If my math is correct, that leaves only 20 percent for training. I don't know if that's straight up or not; in fact, I think it varies by individual and situation. My hunch is that the young blood pumping iron every day to make his high school football squad can probably eat fast food three times a day and still grow like a weed. (Don't do that, by the

**Great spirits have always encountered violent opposition from mediocre minds.**
—ALBERT EINSTEIN

way.) In his special situation, nutrition might only be 20 percent of the equation. On the other hand, if a woman weighs 200 more pounds than she should, the dietary component of her body solution might be more like 90 percent—although she absolutely will need to become more active to start making progress and then sustain it.

That's one way of looking at it. Another is that the diet part of the Platinum Workout makes up about 20 percent of the actions, the time, the energy, and so on that you must take to achieve the final result. And there's another law stating that 20 percent of what you do produces 80 percent of your results. Or in a meeting—the last 20 percent gives you 80 percent of what you're trying to accomplish. Here, you're exerting less energy handling the nutrition part than you are banging out sets and reps in the gym, but it's having the biggest effect on your body.

Yet whether the 80/20 or 20/80 ratio is over-estimating or underestimating nutrition's impor-tance, no one really argues this point:

**Success = training + nutrition**

*You simply cannot get the body you want unless you're eating the right way. Period.*

Throughout the Platinum Workout, you'll find information on how to eat during the various stages of the program (Bronze, Silver, Gold, and Platinum). In fact, the Bronze Phase started with a week in which you didn't train at all. Instead, you dedicated yourself to getting your kitchen in order so that you could fuel your body properly when you do start training. Each of those phases also gives you sample meal plans showing you *exactly* how to eat the way that I do.

Those sample meal plans come courtesy of the consulting nutritionist for the Platinum Workout, Christopher Mohr, PhD, RD. The dude knows his stuff: A registered dietitian (that's what the RD means), Chris holds a bachelor's degree in human nutrition with a minor in kinesiology from Penn State University, a master's degree in nutrition sci-ence from the University of Massachusetts, and a doctorate in exercise physiology from the Univer-sity of Pittsburgh (that's where the PhD comes from). His doctoral work focused on the preven-

tion and treatment of obesity. He has also written a textbook on sports nutrition and articles on high-performance nutrition for *Men's Health* and other magazines.

In order to get into the nuts and bolts—specifi-cally, the do's and don'ts, which is what you care about, rather than a bunch of whacked-out sci-ence—I sat down with Chris for a no-nonsense conversation about Platinum Workout nutrition. So listen up: This information alone can change your life, in part by making it a lot longer and healthier.

**LL:** Chris, I eat oatmeal for breakfast. Protein shakes, fruit, things like that. Explain to the people what the benefits are of eating that way.

**Mohr:** That's great, LL. Oatmeal is a staple of a healthy breakfast because of the nutrients offered. So are eggs, which offer many important nutrients and a lot of protein for building muscle as well. Protein shakes blended with fruit are another great option, particularly for the sake of ease. Any kind of whole-grain cereal topped with fruit, perhaps along with some cottage cheese, too, is a winning combination. You want to combine whole grains and protein.

**LL:** I know eggs get a bad rap, but I actually like eggs. Tell the people why that's okay.

**Mohr:** Eggs have gotten a very bad rap. Studies have shown recently just how beneficial they are for you. Eggs are a great and inexpensive source of "complete" protein, with tons of amino acids. They also offer loads of nutrients such as vita-min A, vitamin E, and choline, which is great for brain health. Eggs are definitely a great food and a staple of the Platinum Workout program.

**LL:** Sometimes I even eat the yolks. Is that cool?

**Mohr:** The yolks are an important part of the egg. They con-tain all those vitamins and minerals that I mentioned. Remove them, and you get the protein only. You also take out the fat, and the fat can be beneficial.

**LL:** Let's explain how we break down lunch.

**Mohr:** Lean forms of protein such as grilled chicken breast and turkey breast are great. Throw the turkey breast on whole-grain bread and you have a quick sandwich to go. Canned tuna and canned salmon are great as well. Mix them with brown rice or whole-wheat pasta. Yogurt is always a good, quick item to boost your protein intake, and it offers a ton of nutrients. Those quick options will be convenient for most readers.

**LL:** What kinds of things do we favor for dinner?

**Mohr:** Similar things to what you had at lunch, but maybe instead of canned salmon or canned tuna, opt for grilled fresh fish or baked fish. Don't hesitate to go with chicken breast, either grilled or baked. And, again, you want some kind of whole grain. Whole-grain pasta, brown rice, and quinoa are all aces. A salad topped with lean protein would be another great option to help build muscle, recover from workouts, and stay healthy.

**LL:** My friends laugh when they see me eating five, six, even seven times a day. Explain why I do that.

**Mohr:** It's great to space out your calories more equally by eating smaller meals throughout the day, rather than just consuming the conventional three squares. So I definitely would like readers to eat snacks between breakfast and lunch, between lunch and dinner, and probably another between dinner and bedtime.

The snacks should be along the lines of a protein shake, cottage cheese, yogurt, fruit, vegetables, and so on. Again, make sure you're eating lean protein consistently throughout the day. Trail mix with mixed nuts and dried fruit is also a great source of healthy fats. These snacks will actually be similar in calories to your main meals. Don't think of them as small meals just because we refer to them as snacks.

**LL:** Let's address the theory that eating immediately before hitting the sack will turn the food to fat. I eat late, and I've never had a problem—at least not since I've been working out the platinum way.

**Mohr:** A lot of people believe that, but I don't. The most important consideration here is your overall energy balance. In other words, if your body needs 2,000 calories a day, for example, and you've only eaten 1,000 by 9:00 p.m., eating those additional 1,000 calories late won't predispose them to being stored as fat.

Having said that, some snacks are better than others late at night. Specifically, you don't want your insulin levels high just before lying down to sleep. So I would opt for a smaller meal—something a little higher in protein and healthy fats and lower in carbs. And these carbs shouldn't be the ones that cause insulin spikes, so vegetables would be great. Some of the fruits with a lower glycemic index would work well here, too.

Also, you may not sleep well if you eat immediately before hitting the sack. And impaired sleep will disrupt muscle repair overnight.

**LL:** Am I right to be eating before I work out?

**Mohr:** Definitely—especially if you're working out in the morning. But eat a little while before your workout—maybe a half hour out—not right before it begins.

Eat something light that can be easily digested and boost your energy: yogurt, a piece of fruit, a protein shake—something along those lines. If you go to the gym on an empty stomach, you're not going to have enough energy for your workout, and that's going to decrease your intensity. You also risk training in what's called a negative nitrogen balance, and in that worst case you can actually harm your muscles more than help them at the gym.

**LL:** And I'm right to eat after I work out?

**Mohr:** Absolutely—right after you finish that last rep, and then about an hour later. Arguably, this is the most important meal of the day along with breakfast. Post-workout nutrition is the starting point for your recovery from training.

For post-workout nutrition, you definitely want carbohydrates and some protein, primarily. Most of the research now suggests a ratio of anywhere from 2:1 to 4:1 carbs to protein, meaning consume 1 gram of protein for every 2 or 4 grams of carbohydrates. It's a continuum: Strength athletes can steer more toward 2:1, and endurance athletes more toward 4:1.

This is the one time of day when you want to emphasize rush (often called simple) carbs, which are absorbed more rapidly than good-morning (often called complex) carbs by the body. That's what you want after a workout, when your body is a basically like a sponge, ready to soak up anything and everything. For the same reason, you want a quick-acting protein.

Drinks and supplements can be really effective here. In fact, many products on the market are formulated with those ratios in mind. Or you can eat a quick, easily digested meal. Fruit, protein shakes . . . Those premade yogurt smoothies are good here, too. And one of my personal favorites is chocolate milk. A study published recently in the *International Journal of Sports Nutrition and Exercise Metabolism* found that chocolate milk was slightly more effective post-workout than Endurox, one of the ready-made formulations on the market. Of course, if you're lactose intolerant, that's not the solution for you.

**LL:** Now, I have hamburgers and red meat once or twice a week. Three max. Tell the people why that can be healthy if you like red meat.

**Mohr:** Red meat shouldn't be a staple of your daily diet, but it's great several times a week, like you suggest, LL. Along with being an excellent source of protein, lean red meats offer a ton of zinc, iron, magnesium, B vitamins, and other nutrients. So cutting them out wouldn't be smart. But you don't want to live off them, either, because they contain some saturated fat, which isn't as good for you.

**LL:** Can you cheat on this program?

**Mohr:** I think cheating on your diet is important, if only for sanity's sake. But when I say "cheating," I don't mean throwing away an entire day eating just junk. If you can keep about 90 percent of your diet pretty clean, you can cheat on the other 10 percent. That amounts to a couple of meals a week, and that's not going to trash your body.

But even when you're cheating, use your head. If you're going out for pizza, for example, instead of having the whole meat-lovers' version, have plain pizza or pizza with veggies. You're still not having an ideal meal, but at least it's not a complete train wreck.

**LL:** Can I drink alcohol?

**Mohr:** Yes, alcohol is fine on occasion. In fact, a number of studies have shown that a glass of red wine a day may be important for heart health. The problem comes with binge drinking. Alcohol adds a significant number of calories itself, and it gets digested preferentially over other nutrients. So drinking increases the chances that you'll store calories you've already eaten as fat. Ever wonder where beer bellies come from? That's where.

**LL:** If I'm overweight, should I cut down on meals or cut down on calories?

**Mohr:** Calories. Gaining or losing weight all comes down to that energy balance equation I mentioned before. To lose weight, you need to take in fewer calories than your body is expending. I'd still like to see that person have

Cats still can't believe I'm hot, I got 'em irate
The **hip-hop boss of the Empire State**
Cats never front on me, they know I drive weight
It's the best that ever did it, **they call me Cool J**
Been platinum so long, my skin's turning grey
—LL Cool J, **"I'm About To Get Her,"** 2004

small meals throughout the day—just smaller portions within each meal.

**LL:** What if someone hates vegetables? Do they have to eat them or can they pass?

**Mohr:** Unfortunately, yes, you have to eat them because vegetables offer so many nutrients and are so good for your body. Find vegetables you can tolerate, or incorporate them into your diet in ways that minimize their taste. If you're having an omelet in the morning, mix in some vegetables and they'll be masked by the eggs. If you want to throw a little Parmesan cheese on top of your vegetables, again to help mask the flavor, that's fine, too.

**LL:** How much sugar should I eat?

**Mohr:** Limit your sugar intake because it just adds "empty" calories, meaning calories with little or no nutrients. You certainly don't want to add sugar to foods like cereal or to coffee or tea.

**LL:** But what about fruit? Isn't that full of sugar?

**Mohr:** Fruit is full of sugar, but it's healthier sugar. Fruit contains so many nutrients that it's not the type of nonnutritive calories you're getting by just adding plain old table sugar to your foods. So you absolutely should include fruit along with vegetables in your diet regularly throughout the day. The recommended intake is five to nine servings a day, and the best way to do that would be to eat a fruit, a vegetable, or both with every single meal.

**LL:** Can I eat dessert?

**Mohr:** On occasion, yes, depending on the type. People in other countries eat fruit for dessert, so healthier options exist. Or, if you're having cakes, pies, sweets, and those types of foods, watch your portion size. Rather than eating half the cake, have one small slice and then move away from the table. But those kinds of desserts definitely add a lot of calories without giving you many nutrients in return.

**LL:** Say someone is a terrible cook. What should they do?

**Mohr:** Well, you can probably hire someone, LL [laughs]. Otherwise, I would definitely recommend buying a simple cookbook containing meals that can be made in a few quick steps. Learn some basics in the kitchen so don't have to eat out every single meal. At the same time, you don't have to be a gourmet cook and take hours in the kitchen preparing every single meal to build your platinum body.

**LL:** If I'm on a budget, what should I do?

**Mohr:** Concentrate on inexpensive foods that still offer nutritional bang for the buck. Dried beans are a great, cheap source of protein, carbs, and fiber. Shopping at fruit stands is recommended for someone on a budget as well. Canned foods and vegetables are a little less expensive than fresh items yet still provide important nutrients. There are ways to eat healthy and not have to rely on fast food, for example.

**LL:** Speaking of which, can I have some Mickey D's and other fast food on this program?

**Mohr:** You don't have to restrict yourself to never eating in a fast-food restaurant again, but make better choices when you do go. Try grilled and low-fat options. If the restaurant offers salad, choose that or the yogurt that some of them now offer, and definitely avoid belly-buster sodas.

**LL:** When people think about fast food, they're not going to think about salads. They're going to think about burgers, chicken fingers, tacos, French fries—all of that stuff. I understand what you're saying, Chris, but let's say this: You can eat fast food—but only when you're cheating. And that's only because we're going to burn it off of you in the gym. If you're not cheating, you can't have it.

Next question: Can people drink coffee on this program?

**Mohr:** Absolutely. The problem with coffee has more to do with people loading it up with cream and sugar rather than with the beverage itself. Coffee itself isn't bad. Some studies suggest it might even be beneficial.

**LL:** What is fiber, what does it do, and how much of it do you need on this program?

**Mohr:** Fiber is a noncaloric source of nutrients. It's actually a type of carbohydrate, and while it's not really digested by the body, it's very beneficial in helping with nutrient absorption because it slows digestion. It also may lower levels of cholesterol and some of those other bad fats in the body.

As for how much you need, the typical recommendation for males and females alike is 25 to 35 grams a day, maybe slightly higher if you consume an above-average number of calories. One piece of fruit contains a couple of grams of fiber, a bowl of oatmeal has a couple of grams—it adds up quickly throughout the day when you're eating the kinds of healthy foods we've been discussing. It's definitely an important component of the diet.

**LL:** Let's say that you're overweight. Will this program work for you?

**Mohr:** Absolutely. Anytime you start following a nutritional program where you're monitoring calories rather than eating indiscriminately, you'll usually lose weight because you automatically reduce your calories. Suddenly you're exercising at least some degree of portion control. Follow the program to a T as recommended, and it can benefit you.

**LL:** Let's say you're skinny and need to bulk up. Will this program work for you?

**Mohr:** Sure, this program can definitely work for you. If you need to increase your calories—again, now you're monitoring your portion sizes, and you can increase them as long as you're working out in accordance with the programs.

**LL:** What are supplements, and are they the same as the steroids I read about in the paper?

**Mohr:** First off, supplements and steroids are two completely different animals, although the media often lumps them together. As the name implies, supplements should *supplement* your diet; they should never *replace* any foods that you eat or don't eat because they never can. They may play an important role in some people's diets, particularly hard-training athletes who need extra nutritional support because of how they're taxing their bodies. But supplements definitely shouldn't have to make up for what's missing from your regular diet. That needs to be locked in and tight.

As far as pills go, I do recommend that everyone take a basic multivitamin/mineral to fill in any missing nutritional holes in the diet. It doesn't have to be anything fancy—just something purchased over the counter at a drugstore or vitamin store will do fine. In certain situations, women on the Platinum Workout plan might want to take supplemental calcium, particularly if they don't drink a lot of milk or otherwise consume much dairy. Older individuals on the program might want to consider taking extra B vitamins.

On the powder side, a protein shake or meal-replacement product can be useful, as long as you're not relying on it but rather using it as convenient source of lean protein and other nutrients. One advantage is the lack of fat.

**LL:** What's the single best thing I should do for my nutrition? Break it down for me.

**Mohr:** The most important thing is making sure you're eating enough fruit and vegetables. A lot of people don't eat any! One thing I've always recommended is to make sure that every single time you eat, make sure your plate features a rainbow of color. The more colors on the plate, the better.

**LL:** I appreciate you taking the time, man. Now I see where you got that PhD.
**Mohr:** Thanks, LL. Anytime.

# Feeding the Machine

While some nutritional principles apply universally, every individual has specific caloric needs. Yours are determined by a variety of factors, including age, height, and activity level. All else being equal, someone who sits in front of a computer all day needs fewer calories than I do when working out while on tour.

The table on page 40 offers general recommendations for maintaining a healthy body weight. Notice that the more active you are, the more food you need and can enjoy—so make sure you get that body moving!

Of course, what matters isn't just how much you eat but also the quality of what you eat. Typically, the plate of a balanced meal should include the following items:

- 1 part lean protein
- 1 part whole-grain carbohydrate
- Half the plate filled with fruit and/or vegetables of different colors

The only thing left to decide is what type of foods should fill up those slots on the plate. The lists on pages 40 to 42, while not comprehensive, offer guidance for making great decisions.

# How Many Calories Do You Need?

| GENDER | AGE (YEARS) | ACTIVITY LEVEL | | |
| --- | --- | --- | --- | --- |
| | | SEDENTARY | MODERATELY ACTIVE | ACTIVE |
| Female | 14–18 | 1,800 | 2,000 | 2,400 |
| | 19–30 | 2,000 | 2,000–2,200 | 2,400 |
| | 31–50 | 1,800 | 2,000 | 2,200 |
| Male | 14–18 | 2,200 | 2,400–2,800 | 2,800–3,200 |
| | 19–30 | 2,400 | 2,600–2,800 | 3,000 |
| | 31–50 | 2,200 | 2,400–2,600 | 2,800–3,000 |

Source: National Heart, Lung, and Blood Institute; National Institutes of Health; U.S. Department of Health and Human Services

# Carbohydrates

| SELECT MOST OFTEN | SELECT MODERATELY | SELECT LEAST OFTEN |
| --- | --- | --- |
| Barley | Corn bread | Brown rice syrup |
| Beans | Corn tortillas | Brown sugar |
| Brown rice | Couscous | Chicory syrup |
| Buckwheat | Crackers | Confectioners' sugar |
| Bulgur (cracked wheat) | Flour tortillas | Corn syrup |
| Oatmeal | Grits | Dextrose |
| Quinoa | Macaroni | Evaporated cane juice |
| Wheat berries | Most ready-to-eat breakfast cereals | Glucose |
| Whole-grain bread | Noodles | High-fructose corn syrup |
| Whole-grain cornmeal | Pitas | Honey |
| Whole rye | Pretzels | Maltodextrin |
| Whole-wheat crackers | Spaghetti | Malt syrup |
| Whole-wheat pasta | White bread | Molasses |
| Whole-wheat tortillas | White rice | Raw sugar |
| Wild rice | White sandwich buns and rolls | |

## Protein

| SELECT MOST OFTEN | SELECT MODERATELY | SELECT LEAST OFTEN |
|---|---|---|
| Beans | Canadian bacon | Bacon |
| Chicken breast (without skin) | Lean cuts of beef/pork | Chicken (with skin) |
| Crab | Low-fat luncheon meats (e.g., turkey) | Chicken wings |
| Egg whites | Mixed nuts | Fatty beef, lamb, pork |
| Flounder | Peanut butter | Fatty luncheon meats (e.g., bologna, pastrami, corned beef) |
| Halibut | Reduced-fat and part-skim cheese | |
| Low-fat/fat-free cottage cheese | Shrimp | Fried chicken and fish |
| Low-fat/fat-free milk | Texturized vegetable protein | Liver |
| Low-fat/fat-free yogurt | Turkey bacon | Ribs |
| Salmon | Whole eggs | Sausage |
| Snapper (red or blue) | | Turkey (with skin) |
| Soy milk | | Untrimmed beef and pork |
| Tilapia | | Whole milk |
| Tofu | | Whole-milk cheese |
| Tuna (steaks or canned, in water) | | |
| Turkey breast (without skin) | | |

## Fat

| SELECT MOST OFTEN | SELECT MODERATELY | SELECT LEAST OFTEN |
|---|---|---|
| Avocado | Egg yolks | Animal fat |
| Fish oil | Margarine (without trans fat) | Butter |
| Flax oil | Vegetable oil | Coconut oil |
| Mixed nuts | | Cream |
| Olive oil | | Fried foods |
| Olives | | Ice cream |
| Soybean oil | | Lard/shortening |
| Sunflower oil | | Shortening |
| Walnut oil | | Sour cream |
| | | Whole-fat dairy products |

# Eating Your Colors: Fruits and Vegetables by Color

Eat a variety of fruits and vegetables from *every column* daily

| GREEN | YELLOW/ORANGE | BLUE/PURPLE | WHITE | RED |
|---|---|---|---|---|
| Artichoke | Acorn squash | Beets | Bananas | Apples |
| Arugula | Apricots | Blackberries | Cauliflower | Pomegranates |
| Asparagus | Butternut squash | Black grapes | Garlic | Radishes |
| Bean sprouts | Cantaloupe | Blueberries | Mushrooms | Raspberries |
| Bok choy | Carrots | Cabbage | Onions | Red onions |
| Broccoli | Corn | Eggplant | Parsnips | Red peppers |
| Brussels sprouts | Grapefruit | Elderberries | Potatoes | Strawberries |
| Cabbage | Lemons | Figs | Shallots | Tomato juice |
| Celery | Mangoes | Plums | Turnips | Tomatoes |
| Collard greens | Nectarines | | Wax beans | Watermelon |
| Cucumbers | Oranges | | | |
| Green beans | Papayas | | | |
| Green grapes | Peaches | | | |
| Green peas | Pineapples | | | |
| Green peppers | Pumpkins | | | |
| Kale | Sweet potatoes | | | |
| Kiwifruit | Yellow squash | | | |
| Lima beans | | | | |
| Mustard greens | | | | |
| Okra | | | | |
| Peas | | | | |
| Romaine lettuce | | | | |
| Spinach | | | | |
| Turnip greens | | | | |
| Watercress | | | | |
| Zucchini | | | | |

**LL'S LIVE-LONGER TIP** Drink 2 cups of green tea every day. It gently boosts your metabolism and is loaded with cancer-fighting antioxidants. The most potent among them has demonstrated 100 times the antioxidant power of vitamin C and 25 times the power of vitamin E. So drink up!

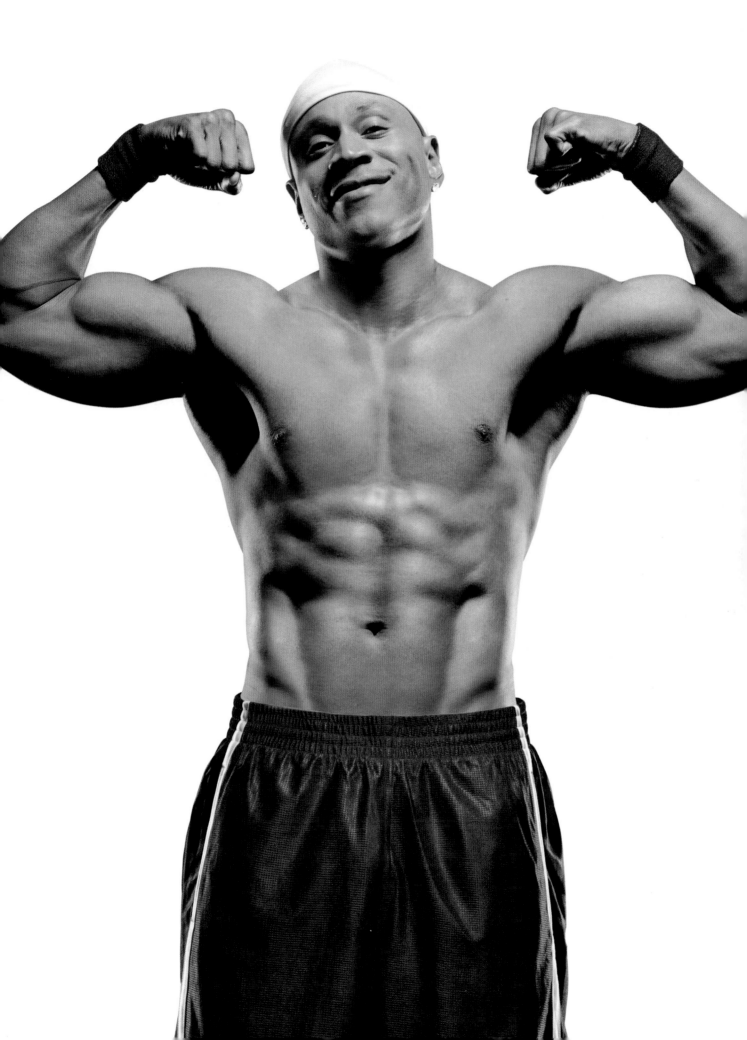

# chapter six

# YOUR PLATINUM MEAL PLANS

**W**HEN I'M on the road touring or making a movie, the best thing in the world is when Scooter sends me my workout and my diet for that day. It's like a road map telling me exactly what I need to do to feed the platinum body. What do I eat today? Well, I don't want to think about it—do you? Like me, I'm sure you'd rather be told exactly what to put in your mouth for the entire day, and then just hit repeat.

So here are the meal plans you need to put your diet on autopilot. Scooter; Christopher Mohr, PhD, RD; and I took what I eat and perfected it for your lifestyle. These meal plans will take you from your first meal on Monday morning to your last meal on Friday night, right before you call it a

**You may delay but time will not.**
**—BENJAMIN FRANKLIN**

week. Come the weekend, you have a choice— either start over again, or use those 2 days to cheat a little, as long as you don't overdo it. (In fact, by the time you reach the Gold and Platinum Phases, you definitely should be keeping your cheating to a bare minimum.) Even if you do cheat on the weekends, help yourself to items such as the Platinum Chili and Platinum Burger, scattered throughout the book. That way you can cheat without really cheating.

The total number of calories contained in these meal plans are estimates for an average person who is physically active, which obviously applies to any reader of this book. If you want to customize your calorie consumption, Scooter uses the following simple calculations.

**To lose weight: (current weight in pounds) × 10 = total calories needed/day**

**To maintain your current weight: (current weight in pounds) × 12.5 = total calories needed/day**

**To gain weight: (current weight in pounds) × 15 = total calories needed/day**

As you progress from one phase to the next, of course, what you consume will have to be adjusted to reflect your progress—maybe a little more protein here, a little more carbohydrate there, a little less fat here. Here's how we'd like you to adjust.

**Bronze Phase:** During this first phase, the calories, whole-grain carbohydrates, and lean proteins are all bumped up from what you're likely eating at present. The additional calories and carbohydrates are required for optimal energy, while the protein helps with recovery and muscle growth.

**Silver Phase:** During this phase, decrease your calories and carbohydrates a bit to assist with fat loss. Notch up your lean proteins a little higher while keeping your consumption of healthy fats similar to what they were in the previous phase. This will help with recovery and maintaining muscle size. There are still enough calories and carbohydrates to provide adequate energy, but they're slightly lower to begin bringing down body fat. The focus with the carbohydrates is on nutrient-dense fruits and vegetables.

**Gold Phase:** It's time to ramp up the fat loss even more. Bring down your calories a tad more—ultimately, you can't lose fat without bringing them down. Don't overdo it, though, because it's important to still provide adequate energy to the body while holding on to as much muscle as possible. Calories help with this process, as does protein, which needs to remain high during this phase.

## THE PLATINUM SHAKE

In a perfect world, all the food that enters your mouth would provide loads of powerful nutrients and a rainbow of flavors. Alas, we don't live in a perfect world. Next time you're short on time, make your shake Platinum-style: high in protein and loaded with fiber, calcium, omega-3 fats, vitamins, minerals, and antioxidants that LL consumes daily to stay in such amazing shape.

Blend the following:

1 cup fat-free vanilla yogurt

1 cup unsweetened frozen blueberries

1 serving nonfat dry milk powder

½ cup 100% orange juice

1 small handful walnuts

Add water to taste.

*Totals: 563 calories, 75 grams of carbohydrates, 20 grams of protein, 22 grams of fat*

—Christopher R. Mohr, PhD, RD

**Platinum Phase:** You really need to make sure you have enough fuel in the tank. Drop your calories slightly to assist with that last bit of fat loss, and decrease your carbohydrates slightly as well. But keep protein intake the same as previous phases in an effort to retain as much muscle as possible. Energy levels may be a bit lower during this phase, but now that you've lost some weight already, your energy needs aren't as high as they were before. So this final phase should be a breeze!

**Diamond Phase:** Follow the meal plans, but reduce your calories by 20 percent. So if the meal plans include 2,000 calories, knock that back by 400. The easiest way is to reduce any four of your meals by 100 calories each.

MONDAY

# Sample Meal Plan

Meal 1
> 1 cup oatmeal, made with water
> 1 fresh grapefruit
> 1 cup green tea

**Veggie omelet:**
> 2 whole eggs and 6 egg whites
> 1 cup diced vegetables of your choice

Sauté the vegetables and add them to the eggs and egg whites as they cook.

Meal 2 (Snack)
> 2 apples with 2 tablespoons natural peanut butter
> 1 cup green tea

Meal 3
> 1 cup strawberries

**Tuna sandwich:**
> 1 can tuna (in spring water)
> 1 tablespoon mayonnaise
> 1 tablespoon relish
> 2 slices whole-grain bread
> Pickles
> 1 sliced tomato

Combine the tuna, mayonnaise, and relish. Spoon onto the bread and add the pickles and tomato.

Meal 4 (Snack)
> 1 serving sugar-free Jell-O
> 1 meal-replacement powder shake
> 1 tablespoon flax oil
> 1 cup blueberries

Meal 5
> 6 ounces grilled salmon
> 2 sweet potatoes
> 2 cups spinach

Meal 6
> 1 Platinum Shake (see page 45)

*Totals: 2,863 calories, 325 grams of carbohydrates, 198 grams of protein, 90 grams of fat*

TUESDAY

# Sample Meal Plan

Meal 1
> 2 strips turkey bacon
> 1 fresh grapefruit
> 2 slices whole-grain toast

**The LL Cool J omelet:**
> 9 egg whites
> 1 cup spinach
> 1 cup mixed peppers

Sauté the veggies and add them to the egg whites as they cook.

Meal 2 (Snack)
> 1 cup oatmeal
> 1 handful walnuts
> 1 cup green tea

Meal 3

**Power wrap:**
> 1 whole-wheat tortilla
> ½ cup hummus
> 1 handful spinach leaves
> 3 ounces grilled chicken
> ½ cup shredded carrots

Assemble the wrap and enjoy!

Meal 4 (Snack)
> 1 serving sugar-free chocolate pudding
> 1 handful mixed nuts
> 2 apples

Meal 5
> 6 ounces lean red meat
> 1 cup cooked brown rice
> 2 cups steamed mixed vegetables

Meal 6
> 1 Platinum Shake

*Totals: 2,763 calories, 305 grams of carbohydrates, 193 grams of protein, 87 grams of fat*

# Sample Meal Plan

Meal 1
   1 fresh grapefruit
   1 whole-wheat English muffin
   1 cup green tea

**Western omelet:**
   2 whole eggs and 4 egg whites
   ¼ cup shredded reduced-fat cheese
   1 cup diced vegetables of your choice

Sauté the vegetables and add them to the eggs and egg whites as they cook.

Meal 2 (Snack)

**Homemade smoothie:**
   1 cup fat-free vanilla yogurt
   1 cup unsweetened frozen blueberries
   1 scoop vanilla whey protein powder
   1 tablespoon flax oil

Blend all ingredients and add water to taste.

Meal 3
   1 baked potato on the side

**Grilled chicken salad:**
   2 cups mixed greens
   Yellow squash, zucchini, red bell peppers in desired amounts
   6 ounces grilled chicken breast
   ½ fresh avocado
   1 cup strawberries
   2 tablespoons low-fat balsamic vinaigrette

Place the greens and vegetables on a plate; top with the chicken, avocado, and berries; and drizzle with vinaigrette.

Meal 4 (Snack)
   1 meal-replacement powder shake
   1 banana
   1 tablespoon flax oil
   1 cup green tea

Meal 5
   6 ounces Chilean sea bass
   1 medium sweet potato
   2 cups steamed broccoli

Meal 6
   1 Platinum Shake

*Totals: 2,613 calories, 275 grams of carbohydrates, 220 grams of protein, 72 grams of fat*

# Sample Meal Plan

Meal 1
   1 fresh grapefruit

**Breakfast burrito:**
   2 whole eggs and 6 egg whites
   1 cup diced peppers
   ½ cup salsa
   ½ cup reduced-fat pepper jack cheese
   1 whole-wheat tortilla

Scramble the eggs and egg whites; add the peppers, salsa, and cheese; and serve in the tortilla.

Meal 2 (Snack)

**Protein oatmeal:**
   1 cup oatmeal, made with water
   Dash of cinnamon
   1 ounce almonds
   2 scoops vanilla whey protein powder

Add the cinnamon, almonds, and powder to the cooked oatmeal.

Meal 3
   6 ounces grilled chicken
   1 cup whole-wheat pasta
   1 cup marinara sauce, mixed with 1 cup steamed broccoli

Meal 4 (Snack)
   2 apples
   1 serving sugar-free Jell-O
   1 handful walnuts

Meal 5
   6 ounces turkey breast
   1 cup steamed carrots
   1 cup steamed spinach with sautéed garlic
   1 cup brown rice

Meal 6
   1 Platinum Shake

*Totals: 2,528 calories, 285 grams of carbohydrates, 200 grams of protein, 67 grams of fat*

# FRIDAY

# Sample Meal Plan

## Meal 1

**Oatmeal pudding:**
⅓ cup rolled oats
1 cup blueberries
1 handful walnuts
Cinnamon to taste
1 cup skim milk

Blend all ingredients with ¼ cup water and refrigerate overnight. Consistency should be puddinglike.

## Meal 2 (Snack)
1 fresh grapefruit

**Spinach omelet:**
2 egg yolks and 6 egg whites
2 cups spinach
1 garlic clove
1 cup chopped yellow squash

Sauté the vegetables and add them to the egg yolks and egg whites as they cook.

## Meal 3
1 orange
1 apple
1 ounce almonds
1 cup fat-free vanilla yogurt
1 scoop vanilla whey protein powder

## Meal 4 (Snack)

**Tuna salad:**
1 can tuna (in spring water)
1 cup spinach
½ cup black beans
1 tablespoon balsamic vinaigrette

Drain the tuna. Arrange the spinach on a plate. Top with the beans and tuna and drizzle with vinaigrette.

## Meal 5

**Stuffed pepper:**
6 ounces 96% lean red meat
½ cup sautéed mushrooms
½ cup spaghetti sauce
1 whole red or orange bell pepper

Cook the meat; add the mushrooms and sauce. Remove the stem, seeds, and core from the pepper. Stuff the mixture into the cavity and bake at 425°F for 40 minutes.

## Meal 6
1 Platinum Shake (see page 45)

*Totals: 2,597 calories, 235 grams of carbohydrates, 220 grams of protein, 88 grams of fat*

**LL 'S MUSCLE-BUILDING TIP** Turns out that whole milk—which is loaded with protein for feeding muscle tissue—doesn't clog your arteries with the sticky kind of cholesterol after all. UK scientists used full-fat milk to double the consumption of research subjects, and their levels of this bad cholesterol didn't rise in 6 weeks.

# ALL CALORIES AREN'T CREATED EQUAL

Those lazy fatsoes who sit home on their couches all day long—their bodies process every calorie as an equal unit of energy. (Hey, if the shoe fits, change your foot size, or at least trim your toenails.) If you eat more calories than your body burns, then the excess will be stored as body fat. Still, you want to make the best choices while you're inactive because some foods are more nutritious than others. Healthy whole foods such as fruit and vegetables are better options than processed foods such as snack foods and desserts, for instance.

How your body processes calories when you're involved in an exercise program (such as the Platinum Workout), though, is different from when you're inactive. The specific types of calories you take in can have different effects on your body, and the benefits and downsides of certain types of foods vary from one time of day to another.

Here are some different types of calories (and macronutrients) that are beneficial at different times of day.

**1. Protein.** Protein is a metabolically active macronutrient that encourages muscle building. (That means protein builds muscles. Big, strong, massive muscles.) For those who are weight-training, it is beneficial to provide your body with a steady stream of amino acids in the form of dietary protein. That way, your body can make use of the amino acids for all the muscle-building and recovery processes that your body is undergoing during this training phase. *For best results, consume at least 20 to 35 grams of protein (depending on your total calories) at each of your six or so meals every day.*

**2. Complex carbs.** These are the slow-digesting carbohydrates found in such foods as oatmeal, brown rice, yams, and whole-grain bread products. (In *Platinum Workout*, we call them good-morning carbs, because these are excellent to consume early in the morning or even for midmorning snacks or lunch.) They provide a slow yet steady release of energy to help fuel your full day. In the evening or later, they are less beneficial because you need less energy to fuel activities at this time of day. At this point, these calories are more likely to be stored as body fat, so reduce consumption of them.

**3. Simple carbs.** The most common example of simple carbs is sugar. It's quickly absorbed into the bloodstream, and if it's not used for energy in the short term, it's likely to be stored as body fat, particularly when you consume a great deal of it in a short period of time. (In *Platinum Workout*, we call these rush carbs.) However, consuming sugar before and after your workouts can give a big boost to muscle building. Simple carbs—sugars—help drive nutrients and amino acids from protein to your muscles to help them recover and grow after they're trained. Simple carbs have their place before and after workouts; at other times of day, they're much more likely to be stored as body fat.

**4. Not-so-fat fats.** Despite low-fat fad diets, fats are essential for optimal body function. Fat is crucial for numerous body processes and is key for the anabolic, or muscle-building, process. Consuming fats also helps promote healthy joints, hair, and skin. While many fats are considered unhealthy—especially trans fats (hydrogenated fats, found in margarine and baked products such as crackers and cookies)—others, such as mono- and polyunsaturated fats, are good for you. These can help reduce cholesterol levels and protect the heart. Good sources of healthy fats include olive oil, canola oil, avocados, nuts and seeds, and fatty fish such as salmon. Flaxseed and fish oil supplements are also beneficial. Consume healthy fats at most meals, but avoid them directly before or after workouts, as they slow digestion and the workout-recovery process, which will cost you some muscle.

# chapter seven
# BUILDING MUSCLE AND BURNING FAT

> Scooter to me is probably the best trainer in the world. And once you get used to him spittin' in your face, you'll love the workouts.
>
> —LL COOL J

**A**LONG WITH offering a behind-the-scenes glimpse at the craziness of a rap tour, those anecdotes from the road that I began the book with lay the foundation for how you too can build muscle and burn fat at the same time, whether you're a man or a woman, from Venus or Mars, young or old, hip or square, black or white, tall or short, shy or outgoing. It doesn't matter! The same basic training and nutrition principles apply to virtually everyone alive. *Our destination was our next gig. Yours is a brand-new body—the platinum body.*

If nothing else, our whirlwind "fitness" road trip proved one point: There are no excuses. You say you don't have enough time to become fit, that your life is too crazy, that your responsibilities are too overwhelming to allow you to shape up? How about having to give a concert every night or two and figuring out ways to train *on the way* from one to the next, all while getting into not just amazing shape but the best shape of your life? That's why I started stepping off the bus and doing roadwork in between gigs: It was literally the only way to get in the workouts. Sometimes I would even do cardio after the show at 1:00 or 2:00 in the morning. That's *after* pouring my heart and soul—not to mention rivers of sweat—into a performance for 3 hours before a huge audience expecting the show of its life.

*Life is a workout.* You need emotional endurance and stamina, for real. You just have to dig deep. You just have to work hard. "If a task is once begun, never leave it till it's done, be thy labor great or small, do it well or not at all." That's the motto my grandmother and grandfather instilled in me. Do it well or not at all. And I've done everything in life like that. Trust me, if you bring that same level of commitment and passion to your current life that we brought to the "Luv U Better" tour, you will have enough time in the day to go platinum with your body. No matter how busy you are—or you think you are—it can be done.

Not having state-of-the-art equipment is no excuse, either. Jonathan Swift may not have rhymed like I do, but he knew what he was talking about when he said, "Necessity is the mother of invention." On tour we often had no apparatus at hand, but we still figured out ways to accomplish our mission. There was no high-tech cardio machine on the tour bus, so we stepped off and ran. The difference is that even when we didn't have any equipment available, the simple things we did were based on the most cutting-edge science available. *That's* what's high-tech about the Platinum Workout: all the information that we've gathered and backwards-engineered to make shaping up simple for you.

The same goes for nutrition. There are a million reasons why you can't eat the way you need to eat for the platinum body, including time and money. Again, those are excuses. We had no time, and you've already read about the nutritional challenges we faced, what with having to stop at roadside diners from hell and cook for ourselves or having to whip up tuna on the tour bus. If we were able to figure out creative ways to eat six healthy meals a day in those environments, so can you.

You also don't need to be a rocket scientist to figure out what needs to be done. Fitness is a comparatively simple endeavor. There are key concepts and terms you must master, but there aren't a whole lot of them, and once you get into this stuff, you'll absorb information like a sponge. You don't need to be able to recite *Gray's Anatomy* (the book, not the show), although I'm certainly not going to discourage you if you want to know what the tibia is or how the nephrons in your kidneys work. When I'm writing a successful hit song, I choose certain notes representing only a small percentage of the total notes available. I take the ones I need and set aside the rest. You can do the same in learning what you feel you need to know about exercise science, anatomy, kinesiology, and sports nutrition.

Finally, even if you have the time and resources to train, you don't have to become overwhelmed by the personal challenges we all face every day. Use being fit to deal with them; don't let them separate you from your most potent weapon. Maximize your potential given your own unique circumstances en route to becoming the very best you can be. I'm going to show you how. If you need someone to hold your hand or pat you on the back, I'm here. If you need someone to kick you in the tail, I'm here for that, too. I've got your back, unconditionally. The point is to do your best to succeed because even if you achieve half your goals, that half will be pretty satisfying if your goals are lofty enough.

At the end of the day, working out is deciding, *You know what, I'm going to do this. I'm no longer satisfied with where I'm at. I'm going to the next level. The next dimension. I'm going to push myself. I'm going to explore something new.* That's the thing in life: You have to keep pushing, pushing, pushing, and then push some more. And you don't stop.

## Breaking It Down

If I had to distill it down to one sentence, here is what I now know produces the platinum body: The human body responds best to short, hard, intense workouts followed by rest and recuperation and supported by a sound dietary program based on eating small meals, consisting mostly of nutritious whole foods, throughout the day.

Sound simple?

Well, it is. I'm not sending people to the moon here. If you read closely, you'll see that I've already broken down the three primary components: training, nutrition, and rest and recuperation (R&R). Think of this as the LL Cool J Fitness CD. One-two-three. Put them together and nothing can stop you.

## Training

The centermost part of the disc, **training**, is also the most fun. I *love* breaking a sweat and feeling my muscles work. Trust me, by the time you reach the end of the Platinum Workout, working out will make your day, as Clint Eastwood would say. As you get rolling, this impulse will only increase. But you have to get rolling.

If training is one of the three pillars of physical fitness, that individual pillar can be sectioned three ways: *resistance training*, *cardiovascular exercise*, and *flexibility training,* which we've already hit. In layman's terms, that's weights, cardio, and stretching. To be physically fit, you must consistently do all three. However, the most important, in my opinion, is resistance training. This is the be-all and end-all of fitness. Basically, when you apply resistance to your muscle tissues, they begin to grow—as long as you're eating enough calories and protein. It's that simple.

Before we go any further, let me hit you with some terms you'll need to know if you don't already.

- A *rep* involves taking an exercise from start to finish one time.
- A *set* refers to any number of those reps (it could be 1, 10, or 100) done in one sequence.
- *Frequency* is the number of times you work out over any given stretch of time.
- *Intensity* generally describes how hard someone is training, but exercise scientists and personal trainers use it more specifically in reference to the amount of weight being lifted (more weight equals greater intensity, which makes sense).
- *Volume* is the total number of sets being done multiplied by the reps for each.
- *Rest*, in a workout context, refers to the downtime between sets.
- *Periodization* refers to dividing your workouts into specific sets-and-reps

schemes to develop specific parts of the muscle. (Think of one of my CDs—they're not slow jams or up-tempo songs all the way through. The material is paced and sequenced for maximum effect. Your training should be the same way.) For example, when training for muscle growth, you want to be lifting weights equal to 60 or 70 percent of what you could lift one and only one time for that exercise. Using less than max weight means you can do more sets and reps. Strength training would be heavier weights and fewer numbers (sets, reps, etc.).

You might equate weight training with building your muscles and cardio with burning off lard, but weights are an amazing weapon in the war against excess body fat. First, you're not burning as many calories during a typical resistance-training session as you are during a typical cardio session, but you are burning calories nonetheless, especially the way I will have you pumping iron. That's the beauty of the platinum approach. I also up the caloric expenditure through the exercises I select—mostly compound movements using free weights, except at the very beginning of the program, for specific reasons that I've already broken down for you. Why does one exercise expend more calories than another? Probably because the harder the move, the more stabilizer muscles that need to be recruited—and that requires additional energy.[1]

Weight training done with an elevated heart rate is also great for melting body fat because it keeps your body burning calories long after you rack the dumbbells. Always remember the Platinum Workout mantra: ***Build muscle and you burn fat.*** To drive home this point, I sat down with the Platinum Workout's consulting exercise guru, Jimmy Peña, MS, CSCS. Jimmy ran the fitness assets for a major hospital chain and several Ritz-Carlton Resorts

and served as director of strength and conditioning at the Baylor–Tom Landry Sports Science & Research Center in Texas. He holds a master's degree in clinical exercise physiology from the University of Texas at Tyler, and his thesis incorporated his own research on the effects of endurance training on size and strength in competitive bodybuilders. Currently, Jimmy serves as fitness director at *Muscle & Fitness* magazine.

**LL:** Jimmy, is it true that muscle cells burn more calories than fat cells?

**Peña:** Yeah, a muscle-bound guy burns more calories standing still than a fat guy does standing still. If you just take one fat cell versus one muscle cell, the difference isn't that great. In fact, it's often overstated. But across the entire body, the cumulative effect is an ability to burn more fat.

**LL:** How big is the difference in calorie burn between cardio and weights?

**Peña:** Cardio burns far more calories. Take a champion bodybuilder, and on his toughest workout day, he won't burn as many calories as a marathon runner or a triathlete does on *his* toughest day.

**LL:** What if you equalized their workout times: 1 hour for the muscle man versus 1 hour for the marathon man?

**Peña:** Still no comparison, LL. The body burns about 5 calories per liter of oxygen consumed, so during identical time frames, the triathlete or cross-country skier traveling across snow is still burning far more calories than someone lifting weights.

**LL:** And in both cases—weights and cardio—the calorie-burning effect doesn't just end with the workout, right?

**Peña:** Correct. When you stop exercising, something called excess post-exercise oxygen consumption (EPOC) occurs.

**LL:** That sounds like a *Star Wars* character. Break it down for me in plain English.

**Peña:** If you're training at a certain level—say, running at 85 percent of your maximum heart rate—and you stop, the

---

[1]*Researchers at Truman State University in Missouri recently found that women who did squats burned nearly 50 percent more calories than women doing leg presses, where the machine stabilizes your body and makes the move easier in the process. Other movements that can also stoke this same dynamic duo of muscle building and fat burning include barbell presses, dumbbell presses, bent-over barbell rows, lunges, pullups, and dips. Not surprisingly, you'll be doing all of those moves frequently in the Platinum Workout program.*

heightened calorie burn doesn't immediately end. Rather, it tapers off gradually over many hours as your body returns to normal. A significant number of additional calories are burned during this window. The exact number depends on how hard you worked out that session.

**LL:** So far cardio seems to have a leg up on weights for fat burning. Is that right?

**Peña:** Not so fast. When you do weights rather than cardio, you may not burn as many calories from fat and other fuel sources during the workout itself or even immediately afterward, but you're still burning extra calories long after the "EPOC window" ends.

**LL:** Because you're building more muscle?

**Peña:** Right on. Remember, we've already established that muscle is more active in your body than fat. So the more muscle you have, the more calories you can potentially burn before, during, *and* after training. And how do you get more muscle? By lifting weights. In contrast, if you have only cardiovascular fitness, you burn most of your calories while you're training. Sure, you get some EPOC effect afterward, but you're not going to be as metabolically active at rest. On the other hand, if *all* you do is lift weights, and you don't engage in those long-duration, high-intensity cardiovascular activities, you won't burn more total calories than the cardio-only guy over 24 hours. So the person who does both, like the Platinum Workout details, has it all.

**LL:** Is this post-EPOC fat-burning effect from more muscle major or minor?

**Peña:** It becomes significant over time. Not necessarily minute to minute or fat cell to muscle cell—that's where you don't see a whole lot of difference. The cumulative effect is what's important. So the key is to build muscle mass to help you to burn fat, and this program definitely does it. You got it all here in the Platinum Workout.

**LL:** Thanks, Jimmy. You're the man.

**Peña:** You got it, LL.

As Jimmy makes clear, cardiovascular exercise is also hugely important. Among other benefits, it helps your body process oxygen and distribute blood to tissues and organs. Examples of the cardio we employ here include walking, running, jumping rope, climbing stairs, and stepups. In addition to burning fat, cardiovascular conditioning can help lower blood pressure, increase "catfish" (a.k.a. good cholesterol) cholesterol, decrease "sticky" (a.k.a. bad cholesterol) cholesterol, and expand lung capacity.

Flexibility is the third pillar of training science. Be sure to read Chapter Four on that subject, if you haven't already. (You're not skipping around, are you?)

## Rest and Recuperation

**R&R** comes next. How easy is that? One of the three major facets of the Platinum Workout calls for you to chill. We're not asking you to climb Everest here—just to relax in ways that are constructive rather than destructive. For example, you can still party. Just don't go crazy.

Rest and recovery are the best supplements on the market. In fact, they're as important as the workouts themselves, especially when the workouts are this challenging. Rest is when your body grows. If you're serious about getting the most out of your Platinum Workout, make it a point to insert some form of relaxation into your day. In addition to the general psychological benefits you'll experience, your body will become more fertile soil for growth. Stress increases cortisol, the chemical that keeps that fat around your belly, in part by countering the positive effects of testosterone and growth hormone. If you don't down-shift when needed, your body won't look and feel as good as it possibly can.

Remember, lifting weights tears down muscle fibers. Only after you've completed your workout will the affected muscle tissues rebuild. To allow that process to unfold, you must give your body adequate downtime between workouts. As a beginner, don't lift more than three or four times a week, never work the same muscle group on consecutive days, and never train a muscle group that's still sore from the last workout.

You also need to eat properly (five or six nutrient-packed meals a day) and get enough shut-eye—at least 8 hours a day. Adequate sleep keeps you mentally and physically sharp for your workouts, and the act of slumber itself releases a cascade of growth-inducing hormones.

*The Platinum Workout is scientifically engineered to enable you to train hard over an extended period of time without getting burned out. The net result is that you'll be able to handle more intensity and more volume more effectively en route to generating extraordinary results.* Throughout, we want to stop you short of getting fully "cooked" from these workouts because the transition from there to being overdone is like a toggle switch.

So when we say to stop, take a day off and, please, rest. Kick back. Chill. Don't overdo it. When I schedule time off in the Platinum Workout, I'm not giving you a day to recover from a drinking binge the night before—it's about recovering from the training workload and the intense demands placed upon your body. *Go out and party and drink like a madman, and your recovery day from that will also be a day when you're not recovering from the training load.* That means the whole process will take twice as long.

It also means you'll be back in the gym before you've recovered. If you shortchange your body by always making it play catch-up, you risk falling victim to overtraining, a syndrome that includes

fatigue and decreased performance. When that happens, your body's energy systems start short-circuiting, and it's damn hard to power them back up. I'm not talking about becoming tired for one or two sessions, because at certain points in the program, that's exactly what I'm trying to achieve in order to make your body adapt. But if you're starting to feel that way for three, four, or five sessions in a row, you're fully cooked, and we need to lower the flame a bit. (See "Don't [Over]Train in Vain," page 190, for symptoms and guidelines on overtraining.)

Essential to recovery—and one of the best ways to avoid overtraining—is sleep. If you think of it as some cosmic joke whereby we surrender a third of our already fleeting lives, think again. No one, including me, can train this hard with insufficient shut-eye. The secretion of human growth hormone, the most powerful anabolic substance in your body, peaks at night, and it takes about 8 hours for it to work its muscle-building magic. What's more, lack of sleep increases the release of that bad hormone we just discussed, cortisol. If you can't sleep, you're probably anxious about something, or maybe you're depressed, or drinking caffeine too close to bedtime, or making other ill-conceived lifestyle choices.

The great thing about exercise and rest is that they work hand in hand. Researchers have established a clear-cut link between stress reduction and exercise, so the very fact that you're working out should make it easier for you to relax and rest when you're not.

## Nutrition

**Nutrition** is the third ring, and we've already hit this hard. Just to reiterate, we're not talking about dietary deprivation. On the contrary: You're going to be eating better than you ever did before, thanks to the meal plans fashioned with great care by our consulting nutritionist, Christopher Mohr,

PhD, RD. Forget about wacky diets that have you starving yourself on celery sticks or eating grapefruit and nothing else all day. The first thing we're going to do on the Platinum Workout program is double the number of meals you eat—in the name of fat loss! Remember, the amazing thing about the nutritional part of this program is that *you're going to be using food to burn fat.*

## Maintaining the Machine—You

Combining training, nutrition, and R&R seems like a relatively simple prescription for maintaining a machine—the human body—that is, after all, incredibly complex. The adult brain weighs only 3 pounds or so but contains 100 billion neurons. The spinal cord weighs a mere 35 grams but contains 1 billion neurons itself. Our body contains 27 *trillion* cells. A sneeze travels upwards of 100 miles per hour. Our hearts pump 40 million gallons of blood over an average lifetime. Ever heard about a lightbulb going on in someone's head? Well, it could, literally. Our brains contain enough juice to power up a 10-watt lightbulb.

But the thing that interests me the most about the human body is that it is truly a manifestation of spirit. When the spirit leaves the body, the body no longer functions. Think about it. Your body will manifest what's going on in your spirit and what's going on in your mind. Think about how you're feeling inside when you grow a beard, when you shave, when you cut your hair, when you eat a lot of junk food. The spirit has a lot to do with what goes on within the body. *Anyone who is healthy can achieve everything I've written in this book. But your spirit will dictate whether you do it.* It's not so much the human body itself, but its fuel—that fuel being faith, that willpower, that determination, that inspiration—which is on the *inside*, like an inner spire. The spires on the top of churches, they go up. In this case, the spire is on the inside. It's the spirit that moves all of this.

That spirit also helps explain why, aside from those mind-boggling statistics I just rattled off, human beings have science, religion, philosophy, technology, language, dreams, society, culture, memory, ethics, self-awareness, myths, abstract thought, and consciousness. The most sophisticated supercomputer in the world is infinitely less complex than our own bodies and minds.

Most of the "software" for this remarkable program comes factory installed in the body. Barring something unfortunate and tragic such as a birth defect, we work pretty much right off the assembly line, or, in this case, out of our mother's womb. Instinctively, our brains and our bodies know exactly what to do right out of the chute.

That's a blessing, needless to say, but it can also be a curse. Because the human body is so miraculously put together, it can easily be taken for granted. For example, just in the United States— the richest country in the history of the Earth, mind you—20.8 million adults and children, or 7 percent of the population, have diabetes. Ten

**LL'S FAT-LOSS & MUSCLE-BUILDING TIP** Broccoli, blueberries, plain yogurt, tuna, olive oil, pine nuts, turkey breast, pure water, yams, brown rice, tomatoes, asparagus, avocados . . . If foods like these are constantly part of your diet, grown organically and cooked to maximize nutritional value, you're on the fast track to fat loss.

million–plus Americans now have or once had cancer. More than a million new incidences of that disease will be diagnosed in the next year, and about half a million Americans will die from it over that span. High blood pressure, a major risk factor for heart attacks and strokes, afflicts 50 to 60 million Americans. No wonder that in the time it took you to read this paragraph—20 seconds—someone in the United States died of a heart attack.

Without a doubt, physical deterioration is partly an inevitable by-product of aging and other factors. But what's a damn shame is that so much of this stuff, and the heartache it produces, could be prevented. Like any other machine, the human body has to be maintained or else. I don't care if you're driving a new Ferrari or a 1974 Chevy Vega—if you don't check the fluids and replace things before they wear out, you *will* stop moving soon enough. Just to cite one example, the chambers in your heart are like the cylinders in your car engine: Keep them clean and they'll keep running great for a long, long time. Don't work them, however, and they rust from inactivity. Use them but don't maintain them, and they get junked up with gunk.

It doesn't have to be that way. I'm 38, and my body fat ranges between 3 and 10 percent. My blood pressure is right on time, too. Without a doubt, I'm in the best shape of my life. I could run circles around a 27-year-old LL Cool J. I would chase him down the block; he would be exhausted. I'd be laughing at him. It isn't an age thing. Just because you're younger than me doesn't mean you're cooler than me, and it doesn't mean that you're more determined than me. ***Dreams don't have deadlines.***

# Get with the Program!

*My Platinum Workout brings everything we just discussed together in one revolutionary program—and*

*you've already started it!* Like the best hip-hop, training the way I do isn't necessarily for the faint of heart. One day I might run the free-weight racks with the maniacal efficiency of a pit bull unleashed in a steak house. The next day, I might go 10 rounds using the mitts, work the heavy bag for a killer total-body workout, or roll it all into a boxing circuit, complete with fingertip pushups and medicine-ball tosses. Cardio might be a mix of medium- and long-distance roadwork or hill runs, wind sprints, and other forms of interval training. Or, to get ripped for a CD cover or video shoot, I might do 2 weeks of 440s, 880s, 100-yard dashes, and hill-climbs wearing a weighted vest. The body ends up thinking, *Whoa, what's going on here? I gotta adapt to this.*

Scooter adds: "Todd could probably do 1,000 pushups if he wanted to, so I realized that I'd somehow have to make the exercise harder. Instead of putting 45-pound plates on his back, I would find a sandbag, because the sandbag can conform to your back, whereas the plates start sliding around. So I would have sandbags measured to 50, 100 pounds and just plop them on his back."

That's not all Scoots can do with something like the trustworthy pushup you first did as a second-grader in gym class. Sometimes he'll have me reach the bottom position, hold it for 5 seconds, and then have me do five ballistic pushups, where I'm exploding off the ground before going back down for another 5-second hold.

We already know how complicated your body is, and it's a lot smarter than you think. So when training it, the element of surprise has to work in your favor. If you repeat the same workout every training session, even for a month, your body can probably handle it without producing an adaptive response. If you feel like your progress has reached a plateau, that's probably what's happening.

Your body responds to exercise just as your brain responds to learning; had you stopped at the ABCs, your brain would be a drain on society. So why on earth would you keep repeating the same workout—the same exercises, the same reps, the same sets—and expect your body to improve continually? Keep pushing your muscles to "learn" more and you will be rewarded with the body you desire before you know it.

## The Zoom Factor

That's why our workouts resemble a roller-coaster ride. They're hard as hell at times but a heck of a lot of fun *all* the time. With the Platinum Workout, you'll move through an easy-to-follow progression—Bronze, Silver, Gold, Platinum—allowing you to invest the amount of time you desire to achieve the body you've always wanted. In 5 short weeks, using the simplest of diets and full-body circuit training, even the most casual among you will shed enough fat and build enough muscle to look your all-time best, a level of achievement shaping the bronze body. A 4-week strength-training phase will give you the silver body, laying the foundation for the full-body free-weight blitzkrieg capable of producing the gold body, a phase lasting 9 weeks.

*Those of you dedicated enough to stick with me for the duration will pass through a final endorphin-stoked stage—complete with jump-rope circuits, weighted-vest runs, wind sprints, and other surprises—unlike anything you've ever experienced before.* At this stage of my physical evolution, these are the workouts I do most often myself, especially when I'm dialing it in for a video shoot. Only after finishing that gauntlet will you possess the coveted platinum body, complete with chiseled abs. (For the ladies and anyone else who wants to try, we offer a monthlong Diamond alternative that's great for shaping up for the beach or a special event. Don't you want to look cut when someone hands you a diamond?)

This scheme is completely consistent with the latest research in exercise science. The best way to build muscle and burn fat is to arrange your training according to distinct phases designed to achieve different yet related goals, including muscle growth, strength, and definition. That's also the best way to avoid overtraining.

## Keep Your Heart Pumping, Scooter Style

In most conventional programs, you do 10 reps of a given exercise, sit around for a couple of minutes resting, do another set, and so on for the duration of your workout. If I were writing a song about this ritual being performed daily in gyms across America, I'd be wracking my brain right now for words that rhyme with *boring*. No wonder so many people throw in the towel.

One of the keys to Scooter's approach is that he shortens those rest periods, or he fills them with light cardio moves until they're no longer rest periods at all because the heart doesn't return all the way to its resting rate. That approach was particularly great for the boxers Scooter would train, where 3-minute rounds would alternate bursts of furious activity with less intense bobbing and weaving. (Ali's rope-a-dope is the most dramatic and extreme example of conserving energy in the ring.) Scooter would try to duplicate every movement a fighter does in his conditioning for a fight.

"Like sprinters and triathletes, fighters are thoroughbreds," explains my main man for muscle. "What I mean by that is they can do everything. They have strength, and they have endurance. If somebody's throwing 150 to 200 punches for each of 15 rounds, wearing 12-ounce gloves, what are his shoulders going to feel like? You have to condition your body and your mind for that."[2]

You can go heavy enough to build muscle and lean out at the same time! In other words, you *can* have the best of both worlds. We take it further still, not only shrinking the rest periods but also having you engage in active rest—say, jumping jacks or running in place—as opposed to sedentary rest: sitting on a bench. *The result is a workout that turns muscle building and fat burning into two sides of the same coin: pure platinum.*

state cardio at the same time you're increasing muscle size. You can't train two opposing systems and expect to get maximum results from both simultaneously. Aerobic exercise and resistance training are very different activities that place disparate demands on the body, which just doesn't seem to be able to give 100 percent to either one. That's a problem for world-class athletes, who need to focus on one activity versus the other to maximize their gains. But Platinum Workout intervals allow you to improve your aerobic base and burn as much fat as possible while gaining strength.

## Interval Training

Another key component of the Platinum Workout program is interval training: alternating periods of higher and lower intensity within a single cardio session. It's a way of training the body to handle more intense, short bursts of activity repeated over long periods of time. Research published recently in the *Canadian Journal of Physiology and Pharmacology* also found that interval exercise is more effective than continuous exercise at incinerating fat.

That's one reason we like it—but there are others, starting with efficiency. During weeks when you're trying to gain size, particularly during the Gold Phase, intervals can keep off the fat and keep your heart pumped without jeopardizing growth, whereas going to the gym and grinding out an hour on the treadmill would be counterproductive. You can't really build up your aerobic base doing steady-

## Join a Gym

One thing you definitely need to do, if you haven't already, is join a gym. When it comes to cardio, I'm all for training outdoors, as our experiences on the road have already made clear. But when it comes to pumping iron, you really need to be in a gym to max it out. Home offers limited opportunities; the gym offers endless possibilities. Sure, you could probably assemble a home setup that's good enough for serviceable workouts. But at home it's almost impossible to duplicate the array of weights and machines found in even a mediocre gym.

The place doesn't have to be cherried out like SportsClub LA, or house machines that look like they belong on the set on a sci-fi movie, or be populated with bronzed lieutenants serving you flavored mineral water on a silver platter after your last set.

[2]*Recent research shows why our approach is great not only for boxers but anyone in the market for a wicked body. A team at the College of New Jersey in Ewing recruited a group of experienced lifters—guys already strong enough to bench their own body weight—and had them bang out either 5 or 10 reps, resting 30 seconds, 1 minute, 2 minutes, 3 minutes, or 5 minutes between sets. These rest periods ran the gamut from circuit training at the low end to powerlifting-type rest periods at the high end. While training, the guys were connected to something called a metabolic cart, allowing the white lab coats to measure how much oxygen they consumed while training. From that they could determine how many calories were being torched. The guys resting 30 seconds between sets—a pace that corresponds more or less to circuit training—burned more than 50 percent more calories than the guys who rested 3 minutes, regardless of whether they performed 5 or 10 reps! The scientists concluded that the rest time between sets has a far greater bearing on calories burned than the number of reps performed during those same sets (Falvo, et al. Effect of loading and rest interval manipulation on mean oxygen consumption during the bench-press exercise. National Strength and Conditioning Association's annual meeting, Las Vegas, 2005). The subjects did have to use less weight as their rest periods decreased, says Falvo, but they were still lifting enough to overload their muscles. At the same time, their calorie burn went through the roof.*

Even a basic gym gives you the essential tools needed to go platinum. It's not about the facility; it's about the spirit. Do you want to make it happen? It doesn't have to be fancy like the gym where we shot these photos. All this stuff is only a manifestation of what's going on inside because that's where we're at in our spirits. But the reality is you don't have to have a zillion bucks to shape up. Look at guys in prison: They're in the bleakest, darkest place imaginable, yet many of them return home in unbelievable shape.

It's not about your gym; it's about your inner location. What gym is in your heart and soul? Put it this way: Entering a garage doesn't make you a car. Likewise, **going into a great gym and having a squeeze bottle and a towel and a nice outfit are not going to whip you into shape. You need to get it on and poppin', baby.** No question.

I also like gyms because they allow you to feed off the energy of others. When somebody walks by, you might just do an extra pushup or something. It's just a good vibe for training. There is a certain type with a certain mind-set who frequents the gym. There's a drive there and often a certain level of success to go along with it. Even if they're crazy, they're *pushing*. And that can be motivating.

Along with inspiration, other gym members represent a storehouse of useful information on exercises, training styles, and workout philosophies. (Just be sure to use the Platinum Workout as your BS meter because not everything you hear will be true.) When I was starting out, I can't tell you how many times I would see someone off in the corner doing some exercise I had never seen before. Some looked great and some looked crazy, but often I was compelled to approach him or her and ask, "Yo, what does that work? What's it hittin'?" Your pet cat at home can't provide the same guidance.

# Old School Is Now in Session

Whether you're training at a blinged-out gym or in the basement at Mom's house, here's what you *won't* be doing during the Platinum Workout: standing on your head, squatting on wobble boards, or balancing a pizza pie in one hand while curling a dumbbell in another during one-legged squats, all in the name of multitasking. Training on unstable surfaces is all the rage now in gyms across America, but it's as overdone as that steak you left on the grill. Some of the stuff I see people doing in gyms is, quite frankly, ridiculous. If you want to teeter around on a balance beam, put down the weights before you hurt somebody, and go train with Bela Karolyi. Better yet, join the traveling circus and perform your acrobatics under the big top.

For the moment, let's ignore the reality that one false move during some of these crazy exercises could break your neck. News flash—they don't work very well, either.[3] Even those of you who do extreme sports like surfing are better served by the Platinum Workout than by lifting weights off balance. If you're a great surfer, you already have superior balance. That's what makes you great at surfing. For you *especially* to be diluting your strength efforts by training in an unstable environment makes no sense. As for improving sports-specific balance, is doing dumbbell presses on a ball anything like standing on a surfboard? Nope. There's a better way to learn how to surf. It's called surfing.

"When you try to combine weight-room exercises with on-the-field exercises, what you end up doing is diminishing the stimulus from both," says Jeffrey M. McBride, PhD, CSCS, an associate professor of biomechanics in the department of health,

---

[3]*Exercise scientists at Appalachian State University had nine experienced lifters squat on a stable surface and then on a ball or disk that wobbled underfoot. The eggheads found that of the two, squatting on a stable surface produced more than 80 percent higher force production and nearly 60 percent higher muscle activation in the quads, which squats target (McBride, J.M., et al. Effect of squatting in stable and unstable conditions on muscle activity and force. National Strength and Conditioning Association's annual meeting, 2005). Fans of training in unstable environments will argue that the point of such training is to increase opposing muscle activity as well as that of stabilizer muscles. Yet the researchers found no improvements there, either, even as muscle activity and force output in the quadriceps fell sharply.*

THE BRONZE BODY

Please believe it, **if the mind can conceive it**
Then the man can achieve it—**you gotta breathe it**

—LL Cool J, **"Paradise," 2002**

leisure, and exercise science at Appalachian State University in Boone, North Carolina. "You're better off doing your strength training in the weight room and your on-the-field things on the field. You need to generate a certain amount of force for strength training. When your force output drops by 50 percent, like it did with the guys in our study, you're not really strength training anymore."

Other research also casts serious doubts about the real benefits of balance-style training. The *Journal of Strength and Conditioning* reported that while young male athletes training on an exercise ball developed a more stable core, that didn't translate to improved performance in their particular sport, whatever it happened to be.

That sums up my take on exercise balls. They're cool for crunches, back extensions, and other core exercises because they improve your range of motion; otherwise, they're kind of corny, and they don't really do all that much. Some of these trainers will tell you, "Oh, it tweaks these little muscles"—yo, keep it real, man. Don't do anything stupid. Just squat with your feet on the floor.

## Lifted Up

I'm also a very big believer in calisthenics such as pullups, chinups, and dips, so get used to moving your own body weight around. What makes these exercises unique is that your own body provides the resistance, not a weight or a machine. As a result, they give you a completely different feeling than weights do. Unlike the aforementioned balance training, they're great for recruiting the smaller muscles stabilizing those big, bad drivers.

However, as your strength increases on calisthenics, you'll be able to do more and more reps without stopping, making them less of a strength stimulus and more a muscle-endurance stimulus—which we encourage at certain times of the training cycle. (You'll be doing quite a bit of that in the Platinum Phase.) Or, to keep body-weight exercises in the realm of strength training, we'll make them harder by using a weight belt or some other apparatus. That's why Scooter will drop a sandbag on my back for pushups or use rubber tubing to make dips harder than they normally are. He's pushing the needle.

So now that you've started the Platinum Workout, keep it going. Don't wait for next week or next month or next year. Life's too short for that. Don't fall victim to what I call the resolution factor, which always fails. *I don't make New Year's resolutions; my life is a resolution.* That's the honest-to-God truth. Tomorrow is better than January, and tonight is better than tomorrow.

# chapter eight

# FREE WEIGHTS AT LAST

**We will either find a way or make one.**

**—HANNIBAL**

**W**E STARTED you off on machines for reasons having to do with the learning curve of your body's nerves and muscles. But now that machines have applied some resistance to your body for 2 weeks—perhaps for the first time in your life—we're going to add our favorite toys, barbells and dumbbells, to the mix. You're ready for it. We know someone as motivated as you are would get impatient spending a full month on nothing but machines, the gym's equivalent of the bunny slope. You know how you feel when you get on the slopes—you're like, "Oh man! A run or two of this is enough—I want to get on the mountain!" We hear you.

As we keep emphasizing, when it comes to training, change is good. Embrace it. Once muscles have become accommodated to the stimulus being applied, they've stopped growing. We want them to keep growing because muscle tissue fuels up the fat-burning furnace. During Week 4—your third week of actual weight training—we swap out one machine movement for each body part, replacing them with your first free-weight movements. For example, instead of just doing machine presses for your pecs, you'll follow those up with incline dumbbell flies. You'll instantly feel the differences between those two training modes—some subtle, some more obvious. For one, without the machine guiding you, you'll have to focus even more intensely on what you're doing in order to remain in the groove during a set. *What's more, without the machine supporting you, the little helper muscles will have to work along with the primary muscle or muscles moving the load.*

In Week 5, we take the training wheels off for good, substituting free-weight moves for the remaining machine ones. Now you're training exclusively with free weights, with a few exceptions, such as hamstrings. (For beginners, these are hard to hit with free weights because dropping your torso down parallel with the floor while keeping your knees and back straight requires good hamstring flexibility without question.)

# Grow Before Blow

One thing you have probably noticed in the program already—and that you might have wondered about—is why, when we have you do weights and cardio on the same day or even in the same session, we start with the weights. We want you to make weight training your top priority because— say it along with me now—when you build muscle, you burn fat.

When you build muscle, you burn fat.

## LL'S PRIME CUTS FOR YOUR BODY

The following 10 foods have such amazing positive effects on the body that Scooter; Christopher Mohr, PhD, RD; and I rate them at the top of the charts, nutritionally speaking. Ranked in no particular order, they are:

**1. Salmon:** Canned or fresh, this fish makes the grade because it's loaded with omega-3 fatty acids. These so-called good fats can improve heart health and mental acuity. Salmon is also a great source of protein.

**2. Walnuts:** Here's another great source of omega-3 fatty acids and fiber.

**3. Tea:** Everyone should include tea in their diet. Studies have demonstrated a laundry list of health benefits, including fat loss, cardiac improvements, cholesterol reduction, stroke reduction, enhanced endurance, and more. For example, researchers at Taiwan's National Cheung University found that the risk of developing high blood pressure drops nearly 50 percent when people drink just 4 ounces of green or oolong tea. Upsize that to 20 ounces, and the risk reduction jumps to 65.

**4. Spinach:** Popeye was right—fresh or frozen, this leafy green vegetable is a great source of vitamins and minerals, particularly vitamin K. It's also a great source of iron, fiber, and beta-carotene, a powerful antioxidant, meaning it's a disease fighter.

**5. Blueberries:** Nothing has more fiber gram for gram. Blueberries are also loaded with antioxidants; in fact, some studies rate them number one for all fruits and vegetables when it comes to antioxidant power. They're also a great source of vitamin C.

**6. Black beans:** They're a great source of fiber and a good source of protein and healthy carbs. Studies have also suggested that their antioxidant levels rank highest among the bean family.

**7. Eggs:** We've already given eggs props, but it bears repeating: These are not only an inexpensive source of complete protein but also full of vitamin E, choline, and lecithin.

**8. Yogurt:** Yogurt makes the cut as a great source of protein, calcium, and healthy bacteria for the gut. Your digestive system will thank you.

**9. Tomatoes:** The magic bullet here is lycopene, an important protector of prostate health in men. But tomatoes are also a great source of vitamins A and C. It's arguably the only fruit or vegetable whose nutrients become more powerful when cooked; in fact, that process helps release the lycopene for your body's use.

**10. Quinoa:** This funky-sounding grain rounds out the top 10 because it's a great source of fiber and B vitamins and a decent source of protein.

# SCOOTER'S *MUSCLE-BUILDING TIP*

Our brains need oxygen to survive and so do our muscles. Generally speaking, the correct way to breathe during exercise is to inhale just prior to the movement and then exhale as you're performing it.

When you build muscle, you burn fat.

When you build muscle, you burn fat.

When you build muscle, you burn fat.

When you build muscle, you burn fat.

When you build muscle, you burn fat.

When you build muscle, you burn fat.

Get the picture?

Doing aerobic exercise first will fatigue you for weight training. *As a rule of thumb, strength training has less of an effect on cardiovascular training than cardio has on strength training.* As an added bonus, when you're pumping iron, your body relies primarily on stored carbohydrates, a.k.a. glycogen, for energy. So by the time you're ready to hop on a treadmill or stationary bike, fat will quickly receive preferential treatment as fuel. You get the best of both worlds. Only that's not all. Training in this sequence boosts your body's natural levels of growth hormone,[1] and growth hormone boosts muscle growth. *This new muscle will boost fat loss, even when you sleep!*

# Week 4: Split-System Training

It's time to split your body for training purposes. That may sound like something that involves David Copperfield, a box, and a saw, but it's far better than it sounds—and really effective at working your body. See, muscles need about 48 hours to recover from resistance training. That means if you did curls on a Monday night, you shouldn't train biceps again till Wednesday night. As you increase the intensity of your workouts, you're going to be demanding more and more from those muscles. That typically requires you to devote more time to the workout, so if you're hitting your whole body in one session, a 45-minute workout can quickly extend to 2 hours. I sure don't have that kind of time. Do you?

Also, the more you get into the Platinum Workout, the more often you're going to *want* to be in the gym. And if you wanted to train your whole body, the maximum number of times you could train on at least 48 hours of rest would be three. If you want to be in the gym more frequently than that—but not for huge amounts of time—you can split your body into, say, upper and lower halves, and train each of those twice a week. So if you're in the gym four times? That's sort of the classic routine. Depending on how far you take your training, you might eventually find yourself lifting weights 6 days a week.

- Warm up for 5 to 10 minutes using a treadmill, a stationary bike, or some other cardio apparatus before each workout. Jumping jacks or running in place will also do the trick.
- Perform three sets of each exercise in conventional straight-set fashion.
- Each set contains 12 reps. The weight you select should cause you to fail on the 12th.
- Rest 1 minute between sets and exercises.
- On the first exercise for each new body part (e.g., chest or biceps or back), start with a warmup set using a very light weight. These don't count toward your three working sets.
- After each workout, do 15 minutes on any cardio machine in the gym. Work at 60 percent of your maximum heart rate (MHR).

[1]*Scientists at Japan's University of Tsukuba had male subjects do a weight workout followed by an hour of cycling at 60 to 65 percent of maximum heart rate. Then the men did the same workouts in reverse order. Doing cardio first elevated GH levels 500 percent relative to resting levels. Impressive, but the weights-first sequence boosted GH levels by 1,600 percent.*

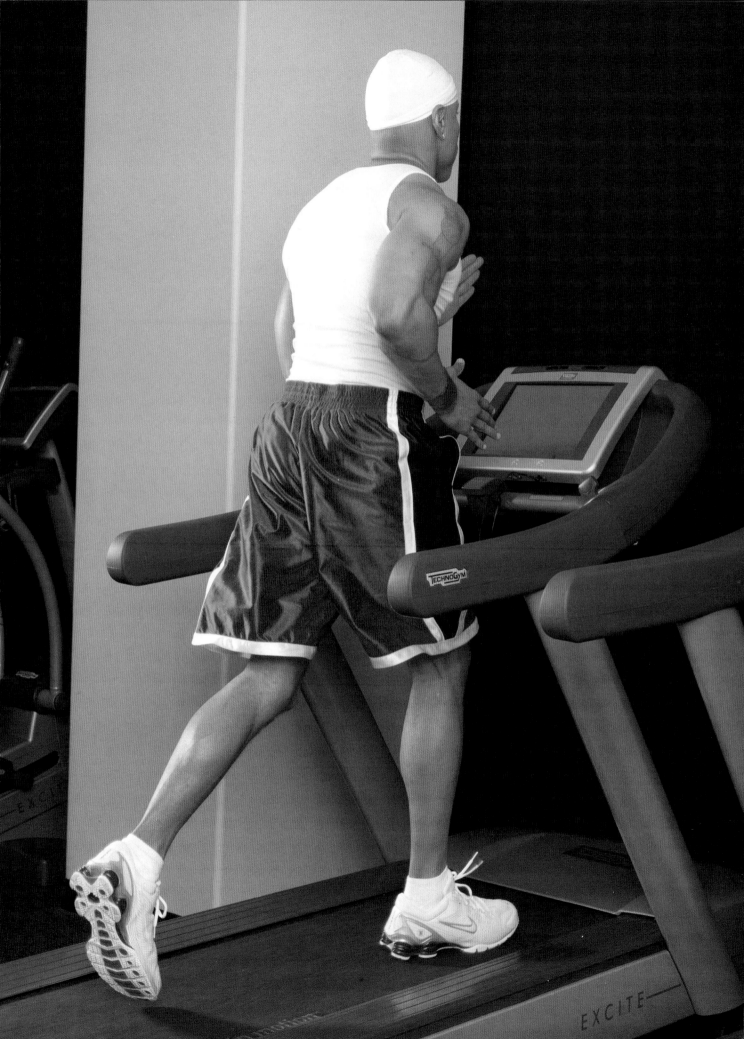

## Monday and Thursday: Upper Body

**Chest**
Machine press
Incline dumbbell fly

**Biceps**
Standing barbell curl

**Back**
Pulldown*
One-arm dumbbell row

**Triceps**
Pushdown†

**Shoulders**
Overhead-press machine
Upright row

*To the front. †Straight handle

## Tuesday and Friday: Lower Body and Abs

**Quads**
Barbell squat
Leg extension

**Hamstrings**
Seated or lying leg curl
Romanian deadlift

**Calves**
Seated calf raise
Standing calf raise

**Abs**
Crunch
Reverse crunch

# DUDE, WHERE'S MY MACHINE?

You may have noticed that the beginning of the Platinum Workout program has you using more weight machines than the later phases do. *While there are specific benefits to barbells, dumbbells, and machines, it often comes down to the simple fact that free weights (the "bells") do a better job of stimulating muscle growth.* For that reason, I've built the core of the program around free weights. Here's a little back-and-forth on the relative advantages of machines and free weights.

### Benefits of Barbells and Dumbbells:

• **Best stimulators of muscle growth.** Nothing stimulates more muscle growth than heavy weight-training moves that involve most of your body, such as deadlifts, squats, and bench presses. Generally, the harder the move, the more muscle it builds.

• **Excellent for stimulating supporting muscle groups.** The bench press targets the chest but also recruits the triceps and shoulders. Free-weight moves are especially effective at hitting more than just the muscle group, helping to stimulate more overall growth.

• **Great for building stabilizers.** One of the key benefits of dumbbells (and barbells to a certain extent) is that they train the little helper muscles to better handle the heavy, less stable moves associated with free weights.

### Benefits of Machines:

• **Good for teaching your target muscle how to work.** When you do transition to free weights for a given exercise and start working stabilizers as well, you'll have trained your target muscle on how it should move, allowing it to stimulate additional growth.

• **Great for isolating a muscle group.** Machines are not just for beginners. More experienced weight trainers may want to better isolate a target muscle, especially on days when an easier workout is desired, when working around an injury, or when trying to rest supporting muscle groups. Machines can also be used later in workouts when stabilizers are taxed from free-weight moves—yet your target muscle still has some work left in it.

• **You're less likely to get injured.** Working with machines at the beginning of a program (or if you're coming back to the gym after being injured) is a great way to reduce the risk of injury. Machines typically force you to work in just one plane of motion, limiting the work your body can do. This is great for beginners but often limiting for more advanced weight trainers.

# Week 5: Split-System Training

- Warm up for 5 to 10 minutes using a treadmill, a stationary bike, or some other cardio apparatus before each workout. Jumping jacks or running in place will also do the trick.
- Perform three sets of each exercise in conventional straight-set fashion.
- Perform eight reps per set. Use a weight that causes you to fail on the eighth rep, allowing you to use slightly heavier weights this week.
- Rest 1 minute between sets and exercises.
- After your first workout this week, do 20 minutes on any cardio machine at 55 percent of MHR for the duration.
- After your second workout, do 15 minutes at 60 percent for the duration.
- After your third workout, do 20 minutes at 60 percent for the duration.
- After your fourth workout, do 15 minutes at 65 percent for the duration.

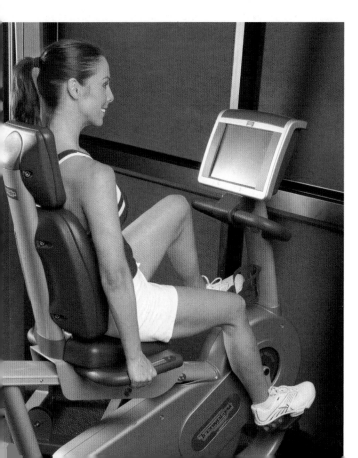

## Monday and Thursday: Upper Body

**Chest**
Incline barbell bench press
Incline dumbbell fly
**Biceps**
Incline dumbbell curl
**Back**
Pulldown*
One-arm dumbbell row
**Triceps**
Dip
**Shoulders**
Seated dumbbell press
Upright row

*To the front

## Tuesday and Friday: Lower Body and Abs

**Quads**
Barbell squat
Dumbbell lunge
**Hamstrings**
Romanian deadlift
Seated or lying leg curl
**Calves**
Seated calf raise
Standing calf raise
**Abs**
Bicycle crunch
Knee-in

# JUST SAY NO TO STEROIDS

When I hear some uninformed person with a doughnut in his hand say that I'm on steroids, I have to laugh. I mean, look at me. Do you know what I would look like if I did steroids? Can you *imagine* what I would *look like*? Seriously, man. I would turn into a freak of nature, lookin' ridiculous, exaggerated, 280 pounds instead of 210, my jaw set hard like a Cro-Magnon man's. Mr. Olympia material. Then those same people would sound all sheepish, like a sitcom character: "Oh, yeah, well, I guess he wasn't. Uh, excuse me. Sorry."

What's happening today is that many young athletes find that they eventually plateau in their natural athletic development. So they turn to performance-enhancing drugs such as steroids. *I'm here to tell you straight up that the risks of steroids are greater than the rewards, by far.* That's not a choice you should make, and it's certainly not a choice I've ever made. My body armor has been assembled the natural way, with hard work and discipline, not with prescriptions and test tubes.

While many of the dangers of steroids have been well publicized, the information often put forth in the media doesn't paint the whole picture. The real risks of steroids often go unstated; the perceived dangers, overstated. Here's a rundown of some of the real reasons to avoid performance-enhancing drugs.

**1. Psychologically, steroids not only are addictive but also exacerbate personality and behavioral problems you would normally work hard to suppress.** Steroids don't cause 'roid rage per se. What they do is exacerbate preexisting neuroses and negative personality traits. If you already have trouble controlling your temper in public, steroids make it *really* hard to control it. People with personalities that already tend toward aggressive behavior (alpha male types) also seem to be more drawn to these drugs than others, helping to perpetuate the idea that steroids themselves lie at the root of the aggression.

**2. Steroid use—especially when unmonitored by a medical specialist—can dangerously shift cholesterol and blood pressure levels.** Steroid use elevates "sticky" cholesterol and can dramatically reduce "catfish" cholesterol, throwing your overall cholesterol ratios totally out of whack. In addition, steroid use drives up blood pressure. While none of these is in itself a "health problem" in the short term, the damage can accumulate over time to cause severe, even life-threatening health problems. Shifting your cholesterol levels can lead to heart disease and blocked arteries, which can set off a catastrophic cardiovascular event. Long-term, elevated blood pressure burdens your kidneys and can even shut them down, making survival depend on dialysis or a kidney transplant. It's easy to buy into the mind-set that you're "only going to do one cycle" and that it won't have much of an effect on your long-term health. But, as with so many drugs, steroids hook you. Many guys like the performance-enhancing effects and start to realize they don't perform as well when they aren't juicing. That's where the above-mentioned health problems come into play.

**3. Steroids will eventually mess up your cortisol response, causing all sorts of health problems associated with aging.** You might have heard that steroids suppress cortisol (a stress hormone) to help increase muscularity. Rather than trying to suppress

**LL'S MOTIVATION TIP** You've got to be really determined to make it happen. You have to do what you're supposed to do when you don't want to do it. There are times in life when you've got to keep going. Now's the time to dig deep.

this hormone, you want your body to respond as nature intended. Screwing with your cortisol levels, as many steroids do, will increase systemic inflammation. Later in life, this has the potential to lead to dementia, insomnia, arthritis, and coronary artery disease, among other problems.

**4. The greatest fear of many would-be male users of steroids is their effect on the appearance of their genitals, but a shrinking "package" should be the least of their steroid-abuse worries.** While steroid use can cause a temporary shrinkage of the testicles and a decrease in libido, stopping steroid use usually reverses these effects. Steroids, however, have a powerful (and negative) effect on your hormone levels. In fact, once you take steroids, don't expect your natural hormone levels ever to return to normal. This means that as you age, you'll need testosterone replacement, not to mention prescription drugs such as Viagra for normal sexual function. Without these pharmaceuticals, your mental acuity, energy, drive, and quality of life will go to hell as you age. You may also find that using steroids will cause coarse, dark hair to grow on your body—not particularly harmful but certainly not a desired effect for most people.

All of which leads to one simple conclusion: Yo, you have to be straight-up crazy to take steroids.

My radio, believe me, I like it loud
I'm the man with a box that can rock the crowd
Walkin' down the street, to the hard-core beat
While my JVC vibrates the concrete
—LL Cool J, **"I Can't Live Without My Radio,"** 1985

# RAP SESSION: WHY FAT ISN'T NECESSARILY PHAT

The Platinum Workout is your ticket to a rap-video body if you want it. Yet for those millions of overweight people who need to become fit and healthy, the washboard abs can wait till tomorrow. To explore what has become a national health crisis, I rapped with a man many consider America's foremost thinker and researcher on obesity: James O. Hill, PhD, the director of the Center for Human Nutrition at the University of Colorado Health Sciences Center. He also was a member of the expert panel charged with developing the National Institutes of Health Guidelines for Management of Overweight and Obesity.

**LL: We often hear talk of an obesity epidemic in America. Is that hyperbole, or is that really what's going down?**

**Hill:** I don't think it's hype to call it that. Whether you call obesity a condition or a disease, it's being seen at levels that were unanticipated and are very, very high.

**LL: I hear a lot of numbers being thrown around, but break it down for me: Approximately what percentage of Americans are overweight right now, and what percentage are obese?**

**Hill:** About one-third of the population is obese, and another 35 or so percent are overweight. That's two-thirds of all adults. Children are measured through a very complex system that's not nearly as reproducible, but what we talk about with kids is 15 percent being overweight or at risk for overweight.

**LL: Is this epidemic unfolding in other parts of the world as well, or is it limited to these shores?**

**Hill:** Just about every country in the world either already has an issue with obesity or is anticipating an issue. Countries such as China and the nations of Eastern Europe, for example, are seeing pretty high rates of overweight and obesity.

**LL: What's the single most important factor contributing to this surge in obesity?**

**Hill:** There's no single thing you can change because it's the compilation of a lot of little things. The way we build our environment influences food intake and physical activity. So the portion size of foods, the fat content of foods, the price of foods being very low, the availability of foods—all those things tend to increase food intake. Technological advances make physical activity unnecessary at work, transportation advances reduce physical activities, and leisure-time activities increasingly promote sedentary rather than active use of time. All these things accumulate, and you can't point at any one as *the* single factor.

**LL: Are Americans uninformed about what causes obesity, or are they informed about it and becoming overweight regardless? To me, it's the difference between knowledge and wisdom. A lot of people know things; they have information. But they lack the wisdom to apply it.**

**Hill:** Yes, I think people know the information, but somehow they haven't internalized it as being such a big problem. Somehow we are almost immune to the statistics, like the fact that 12-year-olds are now developing diabetes. How can you not get upset at that? We know that information and yet somehow we continue to let our kids get obese. With so much information around, it's hard to believe people aren't informed. It's a dilemma with no easy answer.

**LL: What's the outlook for the generation currently in its teens and under 10 years of age?**

**Hill:** It's really looking bleak. You hear people say that because of obesity, this is the first generation whose members will die younger than their parents. Whether it's true or not, it may point out that all the improvements in quality of life over time may slow down in this next generation because of the weight issues we're discussing.

**LL: Has anyone projected what will happen when this generation reaches 30 years of age and their metabolism starts slowing down, too?**

**Hill:** One could speculate that if you get kids developing diabetes in their teens, they're going to have heart disease at 25 and then need a transplant in their thirties. Is that true? Heck, we don't know because we've never gone through this. But from what we know about what happens once you have diabetes, all those consequences seem likely to occur. Before, people would get diabetes in their sixties, and heart disease would follow in their seventies and eighties. Now that we see kids getting diabetes in their teens, will these other things happen in their twenties and thirties? Probably.

**LL: Tell us about the National Weight Control Registry you're involved in.**

**Hill:** It's a group I started with Dr. Rena Wing at Brown University. The registry comprises a group of people who have succeeded at long-term weight-loss management, defined as maintaining at least a 30-pound weight loss for at least 1 full year.

**LL: Are they linked by any commonalities?**

**Hill:** We have identified four major commonalities in how these people keep the weight off once they lose it. First, they eat a high-carbohydrate, moderately low-fat diet. They consistently eat breakfast 7 days a week. They weigh themselves frequently. They keep food records frequently, and on average they do about an hour a day of moderate-intensity activity such as brisk walking. Those strategies all work.

A basehead cleaned up his act
He stopped smokin' crack and took his soul back
Decided, he could find a much better way to live
You know the way—positive
Without all the negative chemicals and drugs
Without all the hangin' with the envious thugs

—LL Cool J, **"The Power of God,"** 1990

# GANGSTER LEAN

**A time line of LL Cool J's career as a recording artist**

## 1982

### ON WHEN HE FIRST ROCKED THE KANGOL:

Oh, man, from the beginning. I had Kangol hats before I made records. Like 14 years old, I starting wearing them around town.

## 1984

### ON HOOKING UP WITH DEF JAM:

I went to a record store, Record Explosion on Jamaica Avenue, and bought a single called "It's Yours" by T La Roc. Rick [Rubin] had formed a production company called Def Jam Productions. I think a label called Party Time distributed them. I bought it and wrote down the address—I still remember the phone number. I think that was the number to his dorm room. I sent Rick the tape, Ed Rock from the Beastie Boys heard it, he let Rick hear it—and the rest is history.

### ON FIRST MEETING RICK RUBIN:

Over the phone and because of his rap music, I thought he was black. I didn't even know that white people got involved with rap. This is just the truth.

When I met him, I was like, "Aw, man, you Rick?"

He said, "Yeah."

I said, "I thought you were black."

He said, "Cool." [laughs]

### ON FIRST HEARING HIMSELF ON THE RADIO:

The first time I heard my song on the radio was "I Need a Beat," which was on a show called *Countdown*. It was 98.7 KISS FM. It was around 8 o'clock at night, Christmastime or something like that, so it was dark already, and I was standing in front of a game room on Farmer's Boulevard. It had rained, so the street was shiny. The moon was out—it was a beautiful night. I was just quietly looking at the streetlight when I heard it coming from the game room. A guy walked up to me and said, "Yo, man, that's your song on the radio." I thought to myself, *I like this. This is me.*

### ON HIS FIRST RECORDING SESSIONS:

We'd do handstands on the subway on the way to the recording sessions. We actually named the recording studio Chung King because we used to get Chinese food from around the corner. That's where the name Chung King Studio came from.

## 1985

### ON BEING A 16-YEAR-OLD WITH A PLATINUM RECORD:

I never felt like I was 16. Do you ever notice how people never perceived me as a kiddie rapper? Think about that. But I really was like [Lil'] Bow Wow and those guys [were later]. I kind of did the Garnett/Kobe thing: I went straight to the pros. So it just felt incredible. I could buy my mother a car, I had money in my pocket, I could buy a VCR, chains, sneakers, I could eat what I wanted. It just felt very fulfilling.

## 1986

### ON WHAT HE REMEMBERS ABOUT THE RAISING HELL TOUR WITH RUN DMC:

Them just crushing me every night onstage [laughs]. And me going on the side of the stage when they were onstage to see if I could get girls. I was like, "I was just onstage, baby!" *Did it work?* Absolutely. Absolutely worked. Without a doubt.

### ON HIS TRADEMARK LIP LICK:

That happens only when I'm anxious or when I'm performing or when I'm in the mix with somethin'. All of a sudden…it's like a tic. I get it from my mother. She does it sometimes. There'll be one month where she's always licking her lips, and then another month where she's cool. That's how I am.

## 1987

### ON THE INSPIRATION BEHIND "I NEED LOVE":

For 3 years, I had been on tour, chillin', datin' all kinds of girls, hangin' out, partyin', you know. *Crazy*, but havin' a good time. Like *Porky's* or somethin'. I needed something less superficial, and I expressed it through my music.

## 1989

**ON WHY A GUY FROM QUEENS WAS RAPPING ABOUT "GOIN' BACK TO CALI":**

That's why I said, "I don't think so." [Laughs] Rick [Rubin] just wanted to do something crazy. I was sitting in the car with him, and music was playing, and I said, "Goin' back to Cali, Cali, goin' back to Cali...I don't think so." And he was like, "Do that! Do that!"

## 1991

**ON WHERE HE WROTE "MAMA SAID KNOCK YOU OUT":**

I was in my condo in Jamaica Estates. I had a room full of guys runnin' all over the place, partyin', hangin' out, drinkin' beer, and I turned up the music real loud and just was rapping. Goin' crazy.

**ON HIS INSPIRATION FOR "AROUND THE WAY GIRL":**

"Around the Way Girl" was just what I liked. I've always been a guy who was more fond of the girl next door than I was of the Hollywood starlet trophy. And I'm still like that.

## 1992

**ON HIS LEGENDARY MTV UNPLUGGED PERFORMANCE:**

They just asked me if I wanted to do it. So I said, "Yeah, I'll do it." They said, "You want to do it with a band?" I said, "Yeah." So they said, "Well, you got to rehearse." I said, "Okay." Went to rehearsal, told the band what I wanted to do, and it ended up being considered this classic performance. I had deodorant caked up under my arms...I was *raw.* I was just doin' what I do. That's what was crazy about it.

## 2003

**ON HIS INSPIRATION FOR "LUV U BETTER":**

It was just true from the heart based on what was goin' on in my life.

**ON WHAT HE CONSIDERS HIS MOST UNDERRATED WORK:**

Sometimes with my music I have to be careful not to be too cerebral because I'm much more of a cerebral person than people think. I like to read, I like chess—I lean that way. It can quickly take me to a place that takes too much thought, which doesn't translate necessarily into a hit record. I don't think any of it's been underrated per se; there have just been some songs that were good, but they took some thought [from listeners], and that's not always great from a commercial standpoint.

**ON HIS FAVORITE SONG OF HIS:**

Probably "Doin' It." I just like that song.

## 2006

**ON HIS BEST MEMORY FROM THE RECENTLY RELEASED TODD SMITH CD:**

The song I did with Mary Mary for me is a real great song. That's a hot song. If that song was in heavy rotation, I think it would really do well.

**ON HIS ROLE AS ONE OF RAP'S ELDER STATESMEN:**

I've been making music a long time, but chronologically, I'm not old. God willing, I still have a lot I want to do in terms of just growing my life. I want to maximize everything that's inside of me, get every dream out of me.

## 2009?

**ON WHETHER INDUCTION INTO THE ROCK 'N' ROLL HALL OF FAME WOULD BE IMPORTANT TO HIM:**

Yeah. Absolutely. That would be great. I would love that. The Rock 'n' Roll Hall of Fame? Oh, man. That would be incredible. The Rock 'n' Roll *Hall of Fame*? That's like stupid, right? You can't get any better than that. That would be crazy.

**Benefits achievable over the next 5 weeks (10 weeks since you started the Platinum Workout):**

**40** percent **INCREASE IN STRENGTH**
while maintaining muscular and cardiovascular endurance

**PROTRUDING BICEPS** and **CHEST**;
**SHAPELIER GLUTES** for women

**50** percent increase in **ENERGY LEVELS**
A **TIGHTER WAISTLINE** for all

phase two
# THE SILVER BODY

# chapter nine

# DESCENDING SETS = RISING STRENGTH

**S**O YOU'VE completed the Bronze Phase. Congrats. You've already accomplished a lot—bronze in the Olympics is nothing to sneeze at. Your body has now passed through what exercise scientists refer to as *anatomical adaptation*, which just means that your muscles, tendons, and ligaments should be strong enough for you to train hard without injuring yourself. What's more, any muscle imbalances evident when you began the program should have been corrected by now. Plus, you've laid down some much-needed muscle tissue. Add that all up and you've built a solid foundation, which will allow you to go balls to the wall when necessary.

*The next 5 weeks are devoted to making you stronger, with continued attention paid to adding muscle and sus-*

**Be ye strengthened by the renewing of your mind.**
—GOD'S WORD

*taining the endurance you've already developed.* What you get with muscle growth is increased size, but that new muscle doesn't have its full strength built into it yet. Think of it as "young" muscle. It needs to mature, and to mature, it needs to strengthen. To do that, we go in the opposite direction now: heavier weights. But because the load is heavier, you have to do fewer reps. Those two elements are like a seesaw; as one goes up, the other has to go down.

So over the course of an exercise in this phase, reps will descend from eight down to four, with that last set followed immediately on occasion by pushups or some other body-weight blaster. Workouts for the big body parts will be interspersed with abdominal circuits and interval cardio—the relentless fat burn continues. Then the weights drop, the reps rise, and all-new exercises are done back-to-back with no rest in between, a Joe Weider invention called supersetting.

Why do fewer reps when you're trying to get stronger? In fact, shouldn't the opposite be true? Seems like more reps equal more strength. Actually, no. When we ask you to do fewer reps than you've done before, it offers the opportunity to go heavier. After all, you should be able to use more weight for four reps than you could use for eight. In turn, these heavier loads apply greater stress and tension to the muscle than lighter weights do. Think about going to the grocery store: Would your muscles strain more and work harder if you lifted one bag or five? The same goes for lifting heavier weights. Increasing the tension on muscle triggers processes that accelerate growth as your muscles adapt to their new challenges.

Beginners, if this seems early to be entering a strength phase, trust me: Your muscles have to get stronger *before* they get bigger. Only then can you overload the fibers enough to truly break them down and make them grow. To use a baseball analogy, you can't leave your foot on first when trying to steal second. And when you talk about strength, rep range is of paramount importance. Although a few of the sets in this phase (the eights) technically fall at the low end of muscle-growth training, most of the rep schemes you'll encounter here will say "strength" to your muscle cells—and those cells will respond big time. Don't worry if you can't use massive weight for your sets of four; use what causes you to fail at the number given, even if it's a little lighter than what the Incredible Hulk on the bench next to you is hoisting overhead. Rep range rules.

Best of all, we promise to sustain your current endurance levels during a strength-training phase.[1]

# Weeks 6 and 7: The Strength Phase, Part I

- Warm up for 5 to 10 minutes using a treadmill, a stationary bike, or some other cardio apparatus before each workout. Jumping jacks or running in place will also do the trick.
- Rest 1½ minutes between sets and exercises, except as noted.
- Try to increase your poundages at least slightly from Week 6 to 7.

## Monday

| EXERCISE | SETS | REPS |
|---|---|---|
| **Chest:** | | |
| Dumbbell bench press | 3 | 8, 6, 4* |
| Incline barbell bench press | 3 | 8, 6, 4† |
| **Arms:** | | |
| Standing barbell curl | 3 | 6 |
| Incline dumbbell curl | 2 | 6 |
| Dip (narrow grip) | 2 | 8 |
| Pushdown | 3 | 6 |
| **Abs:** | | |
| Hanging knee raise | 2 | 10, 15 |
| Knee-in | 2 | 10, 15 |

**Interval cardio:**

Alternate 1 minute of slow jogging at 55 percent of maximum heart rate (MHR) with 1 minute of running at 70 percent of MHR for 12 minutes total.

*Superset final set with pushups with your feet elevated on a bench, done to failure.

†Superset final set with pushups done to failure.

[1]The white lab coats from Louisiana Tech found in a study that powerlifters, who avoid cardio like vampires avoid tanning salons, nonetheless had VO$_2$ max measurements similar to those of endurance athletes. (T.P. Carson. Absolute and relative physiological measures of collegiate power lifters. National Strength and Conditioning Association's annual meeting, Las Vegas, 2005.) VO$_2$ max measures the ability to consume oxygen for conversion into energy. The greater your VO$_2$ max, the higher your fitness level.

# Tuesday

| EXERCISE | SETS | REPS |
|---|---|---|
| Barbell squat | 4 | 10, 8, 6, 4 |
| Leg press (unilateral) | 2 | 8 |
| Lying leg curl | 3 | 8, 6, 4 |
| Romanian deadlift | 3 | 10 |

# Wednesday

Steady-state cardio: Do 30 minutes on any piece of cardio equipment at 65 percent of MHR.

# Thursday

| EXERCISE | SETS | REPS |
|---|---|---|
| **Shoulders:** | | |
| Seated dumbbell press | 3 | 8, 6, 4 |
| Bent-over lateral raise | 3 | 8, 6, 6 |
| Dumbbell lateral raise | 2 | 8, 8 |
| **Scooter's ab circuit no. 1:‡** | | |
| 1. Situp | 2 | 15 |
| 2. Crunch | 2 | 15 |
| 3. Jackknife | 2 | 15 |
| **Triceps** | | |
| *Superset:* | | |
| 1. Skull-crusher | 2 | 8, 6, 6 |
| 2. Dip | 2 | 8, 6, 6 |
| Pushdown | 2 | 15 |

‡Don't rest until you've done all three ab moves consecutively. Then rest 1 minute and repeat until you've done the required sets.

# Friday

| EXERCISE | SETS | REPS |
|---|---|---|
| **Back:** | | |
| Pullup | 3 | To failure |
| Bent-over barbell row | 3 | 8, 6, 4 |
| Seated cable row | 3 | 8, 6, 4 |

**Interval cardio:**

Alternate 1 minute of jogging at 55 percent of MHR with 1 minute of running at 70 percent of MHR for 25 minutes total.

# Saturday

Active rest

# Sunday

Active rest

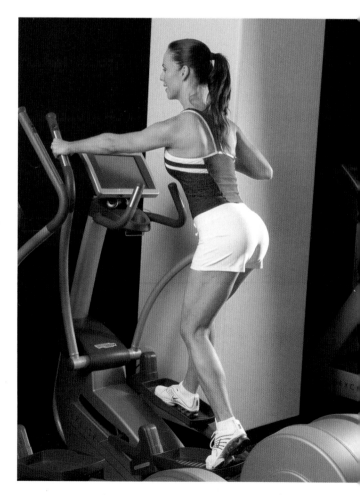

# Weeks 8 and 9:
# The Strength Phase, Part II

- Warm up for 5 to 10 minutes using a treadmill, a stationary bike, or some other cardio apparatus before each workout. Jumping jacks or running in place will also do the trick.
- Rest 2 minutes between all sets and exercises.
- Try to increase your poundage at least slightly from Weeks 8 to 9.

## Monday

| EXERCISE | SETS | REPS |
|---|---|---|
| **Chest:** | | |
| Incline barbell bench press | 3 | 5 |
| Weighted dip (wide grip) | 3 | 5 |
| *Superset:* | | |
| 1. Pushup (feet elevated) | 1 | to failure |
| 2. Incline dumbbell fly | 1 | 15 |

**Interval cardio:**

Alternate 30 seconds of sprinting at 90 to 95 percent of MHR with 1 minute of jogging at 50 percent of MHR for 30 minutes total.

## Tuesday

| EXERCISE | SETS | REPS |
|---|---|---|
| Pullup | 3 | 5 |
| Seated cable row | 3 | 5 |
| Bent-over barbell row | 2 | 15 |
| **Scooter's abs circuit no. 2:*** | | |
| 1. Machine or rope crunch | 3 | 15–20 |
| 2. Hanging knee raise | 3 | 15–20 |
| 3. Knee-in | 3 | 15–20 |

*Don't rest until you've done all three ab moves consecutively. Then rest 1 minute and repeat until you've done the required sets.

## Wednesday

Cardio: Do 35 minutes on a cross-trainer at 65 to 75 percent of MHR.

## Thursday

| EXERCISE | SETS | REPS |
|---|---|---|
| Standing barbell curl | 3 | 5 |
| Dip (close grip) | 3 | 5 |
| Preacher curl | 3 | 5 |
| Pushdown | 3 | 10 |
| **Scooter's ab circuit no. 3:†** | | |
| Reverse crunch | 2 | 15 |
| Decline situp | 2 | 15 |
| Knee-in | 2 | 15 |

†Do these ab moves consecutively. Rest 1 minute. Repeat one more time for two sets total.

## Friday

| EXERCISE | SETS | REPS |
|---|---|---|
| Leg press | 3 | 5 |
| Leg extension | 3 | 5 |
| Lying leg curl | 3 | 5 |
| Standing calf raise | 3 | 5 |
| Seated barbell press | 3 | 5 |

**Interval cardio:**

Alternate 30 seconds of sprinting at 90 to 95 percent of MHR with 1 minute of jogging at 50 percent of MHR for 20 minutes total.

## Saturday

Active rest

## Sunday

Active rest

# Week 10: Active Rest

The blow-and-go style of training that Scooter Pie and I employ for ourselves and advocate for you puts intense pressure on the human body, from the lungs that need to suck in all of that air to the frame that must weather all of that pounding. That's why our program works wonders—and that's why you need to shut things down, or at least throttle them back, now and again. Your entire neuromuscular system needs downtime on occasion. This includes, but isn't limited to, your central nervous system, skeleton, muscles, and the tendons and joints that connect them. Oh, and your brain needs R&R just as much as your body does. Mental fatigue can develop gradually over the long term, but when it finally arrives in force, it can knock you out like an Ali right hook.

*Bottom line: Your mind and body alike just need a chance to shut down and reboot once in a while.*

Specifically, every 10th week or so of training should be devoted to something called active rest—and here we are, at Week 10. Active rest sounds like an oxymoron, but it just means that while we don't want you training balls to the wall this week, like you have been for the past 2 months or so, we don't want you sitting on the sofa killing six-packs, either. Moderate activity is the watchword here. Normally, when we train you in the Platinum Workout, you're *working*, without question. This week should feel more like play.

No need to make it overly programmed; that would defeat the whole purpose of downshifting. Maybe go to the gym once or twice this week, but improvise a fun workout using significantly lighter weights and less volume than you have used previ-

They **pay me so much** it's hard for them to swallow
When you got 'em by the balls, their hearts and minds follow
**Pay yourself first**, that's one of my main mottos
Picture Bill Gates on the block dodgin' hollows
—LL Cool J, **"Shake It Baby,"** 2004

## RAP SESSION: THE NEW SCIENCE OF SIZE

Lifting a hunk of metal from Point A to Point B might seem as simple as "See Spot Train," but as the Platinum Workout suggests, there's a lot more to it than that. To get a handle on the latest research developments in strength training, I rapped with one of the leading experts in the field, David R. Pearson, PhD, CSCS. Dr. Pearson is an associate professor of physical education at Ball State University in Muncie, Indiana, as well as the director of that school's nationally renowned Strength Research Laboratory. He also serves on the editorial advisory board for *Men's Health* magazine.

**LL: In terms of research into resistance training, what's the most important thing we know today that we didn't know 10 years ago?**

**Pearson:** The biggest insight that we now have is periodization. We now understand a plan by which muscle is most efficiently strengthened. We argued for years about the most efficient way to train muscle, and now we know: going from hypertrophy training to strength training and then on to training for power and performance. Nearly everyone agrees with this, from sports coaches to exercise scientists. Secondly, I think we have a much better understanding of the importance of nutrition for muscle than we did 10 years ago.

**LL: Over time, are we learning that resistance training is more or less important for the body than previously thought?**

**Pearson:** Oh, there's no question—health professionals right on through to personal trainers have an ever-increasing understanding of the importance of strength training. Look at it this way: It's wonderful to have a cardiovascular base, but if you're too weak to get out of a chair, you're not going to be able to use it. So we've got to reach the point where people see the benefits of cardiovascular fitness *and* muscular fitness. This is even more important as we age because the primary reason we contract diseases is inactivity, and that comes from getting weaker and weaker.

**LL: We usually think of research as being esoteric,** but are there lessons you've taken from the laboratory straight to the gym yourself?

**Pearson:** I'm an applied exercise physiologist, so just about every research project that I've done has originated with a problem I encountered in the gym. In that regard, I work in the opposite direction of traditional researchers. My own personal research has focused on supplementation and nutrition in athletes. The types of research projects that I've been involved with that have made the greatest difference for me personally have concerned making sure the body is properly fed before training it.

**LL: Other than supplementation and nutrition, what has your own research focused on?**

**Pearson:** One of the things I'm doing is trying to look at ways that we can better train the military, especially the National Guard, for its active role in warfare. In many cases, we're taking people off an 8-to-5 job and throwing them into a very physical situation for which their body hasn't had time to prepare. What's more, the minimum weight of their gear is 70 pounds. Imagine you've signed up with the National Guard, your name is called up, and within a month, you're engaged in combat with an extra 70 pounds on your back. It's something that's going to have to be dealt with long-term because the National Guard will likely be involved in the protection of the country for the foreseeable future.

**LL: Get out your crystal ball: What's the most intriguing development on the horizon in resistance-training research?**

**Pearson:** There is still an awful lot of work to be done in the areas of nutrition and hydration. If we're going to crack this steroid problem, it's going to come though advancements in nutrition and hydration more than anything else. If we're going to convince the 15-year-old of today not to use steroids to achieve a particular level of improvement, we're going to have to show him other ways of achieving significant performance goals. My personal guess is that it's going to come through nutrition and hydration, as opposed to some new type of training. Progressive resistance training has been around since the Greeks invented the Olympics, so I don't know that I'm expecting it to change significantly.

ously in the Platinum Workout. Mess around a little. One or two other days, maybe go for a bike ride or hike, or play a leisurely game of tennis with a friend, or run some stairs—again, taking it at a more leisurely pace than our workouts normally demand. You've earned a break.

Rather than backpedaling, your body will probably grow more during this hard-earned active-rest week than it did over the preceding 2 to 4 weeks. You're finally giving your body the chance to manifest a lot of the gains you've stimulated through hard training and sound eating. Speaking of which, no need to take a break from eating the platinum way

during active rest. Cheat days are already baked into the cake, no pun intended, and we don't want you turning this into a cheat *week*. Because your body likely will experience a growth spurt, make sure it has the nutritional blocks it needs to build muscle.

After spending a week in active-rest mode, resume the program when noted, without delay. Don't backslide. If 1 week turns into 10 days or 2 weeks, you're a bump in the road or two away from falling off the wagon. Scoots and I need you to stay onboard if we're going to take you platinum.

By the time Week 11 starts, you should be loaded for bear.

## THE PLATINUM CHILI

Chili is delicious, inexpensive, and simple to make. Nothing tastes as much like home cooking as a nice potful. In fact, it's a staple for Cool J and his crew when they're on the road.

The Platinum version warrants the adjective "perfect" because the ground meat offers protein, zinc, and iron; the tomato sauce provides a powerful nutrient called lycopene that has been shown to protect prostate health; and the onion is loaded with powerful antioxidants of its own.

Follow these instructions:

**1.** Start off with some lean meat (90% lean or even higher).

**2.** Heat 1 tablespoon oil in a large pot over medium heat.

**3.** Add 1 whole chopped onion, 3 tablespoons chili powder, and 3 tablespoons cumin powder.

**4.** Stir occasionally so that the onion doesn't burn.

**5.** Add 1 pound ground meat and cook until no longer pink (about 10 minutes).

**6.** Add 3 (28-ounce) cans crushed tomatoes and 1 (28-ounce) can whole tomatoes.

**7.** Stir and continue to heat for approximately 60 minutes.

**8.** Add additional seasoning if desired, including salt and pepper.

—Christopher R. Mohr, PhD, RD

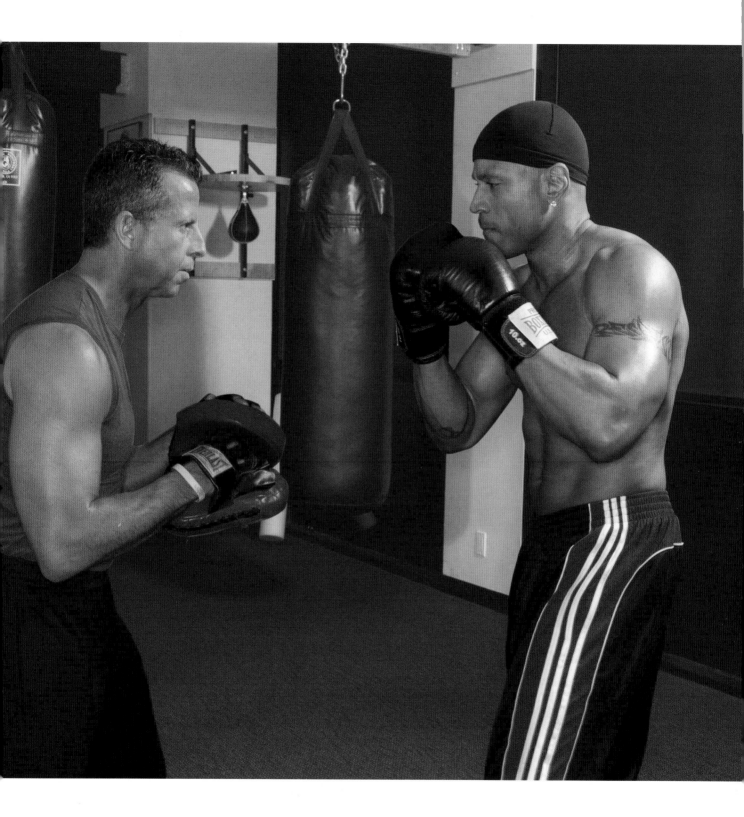

# chapter ten
# THE PLATINUM EXERCISES

**O**NCE YOU decide to work out, you can choose from a list of exercises that is nearly endless. In fact, Arnold Schwarzenegger devoted an entire encyclopedia to them. Scooter "MacGyver" Honig and I like to tinker and experiment by nature, so we've not only tried 90 percent of Arnold's moves but we've also invented a bunch more on our own for good measure.

In the Platinum Workout, though, we've combined our experience and knowledge to narrow down this vast array. That's because beginners to the iron game, especially, should focus on building a great foundation. In our selection process, we relied first and foremost on compound movements because they bring into play a lot of secondary muscles to assist the main movers: chest, back, and quads. You want to hit the beach and flex your locked-and-loaded guns? Not so fast. Focus on the big picture, which is your entire body, not just selected regions, which are body parts. When we do ask you to perform so-called isolation move-

**Quality means doing it right when nobody is looking.**

**—HENRY FORD**

ments, they'll come after "bigger" moves 9 times out of 10 at least.

The reason this variety works well for me is because I become used to things quickly. I have to switch it up constantly. It keeps me from becoming bored. It's adventurous. I can always find a way to get sore again. It sounds weird, but it's not easy. Like right now, I'd have to do a couple hundred pushups just to get sore. So I love switchin' it up. I love addressing it in different ways. That's why I do all kinds of stuff.

Get used to this approach. Embrace it. In life, not just in the gym, it's good to switch it up. Trust me, if you don't like change, you'll like irrelevance even less. Word up.

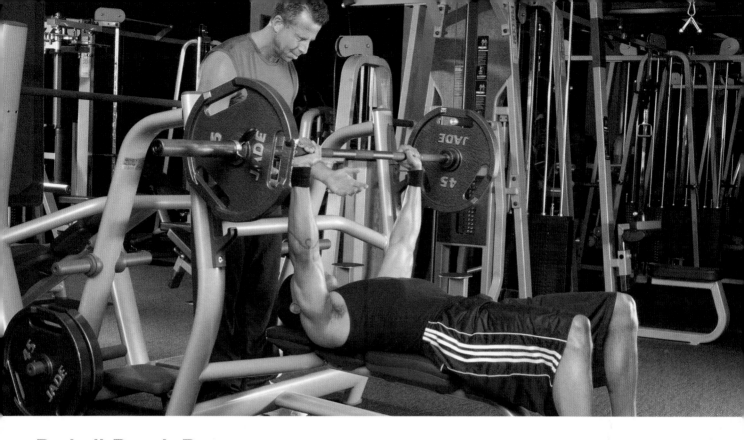

## Barbell Bench Press

1. Lie faceup with your back flat against the pad and your feet planted on the floor. Take several deep breaths.

2. Unrack the bar and raise it above you at arms' length. This is the start position.

3. Lower the bar at a three-count until it touches your upper chest. Inhale during the descent.

4. Without "bouncing" off the bottom, push the weight back up at a 2-count to the start position. Exhale during the ascent, and don't lock out your arms at the top.

5. Make sure your glutes remain on the bench, your eyes stay trained on the ceiling, and your wrists stay straight at all times.

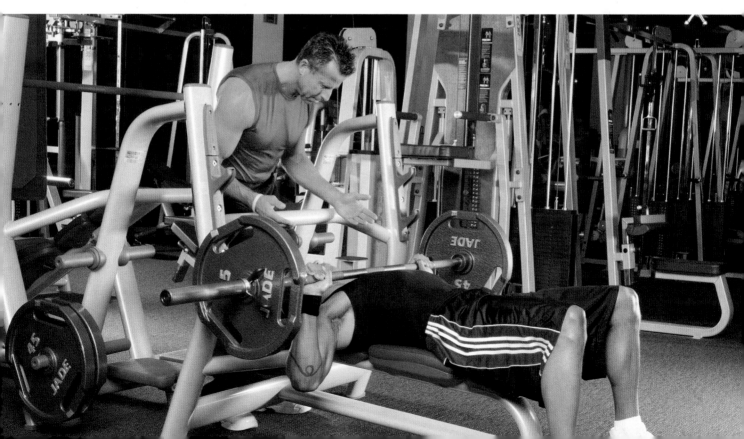

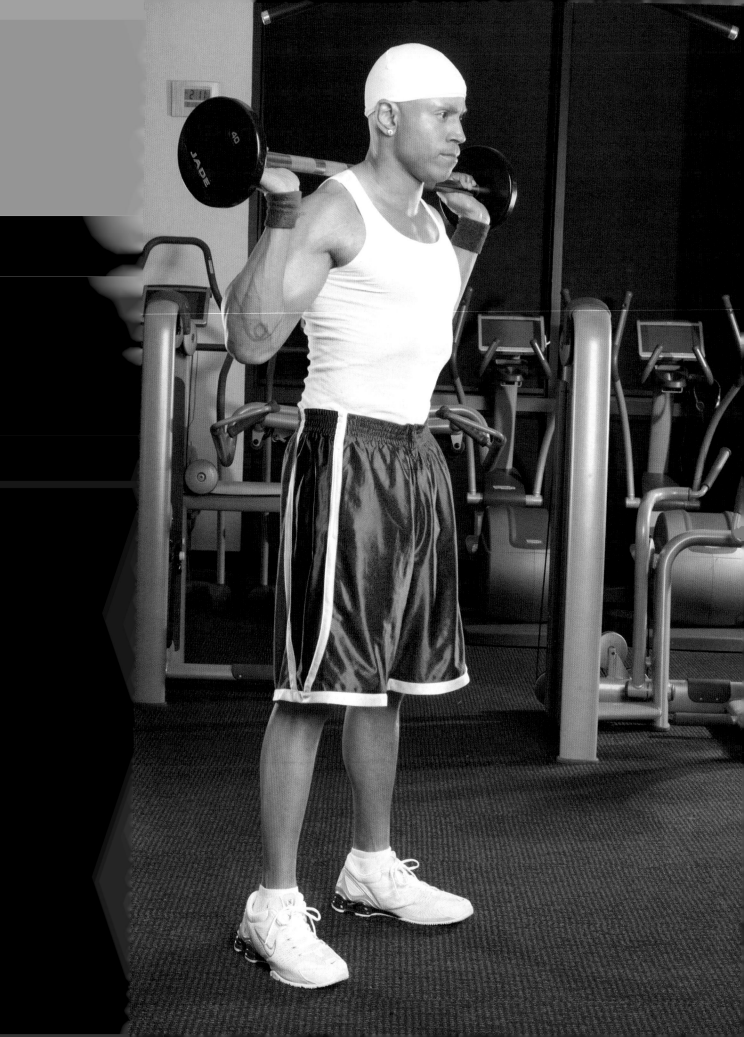

# Barbell Squat

1. Step under the bar in a squat rack with your feet parallel to each other, shoulder-width apart. Grasp the bar with an overhand grip so it rests across your traps.

2. Step back and stand with chest high, shoulder blades squeezed back, gaze fixed forward. This is the start position.

3. Bend your knees as if sitting down in a chair, making sure that your knees stay aligned with your feet, until your thighs are parallel with the floor.

4. Push up through your feet without bouncing to return to the start position. Avoid locking out your knees at the top of the movement.

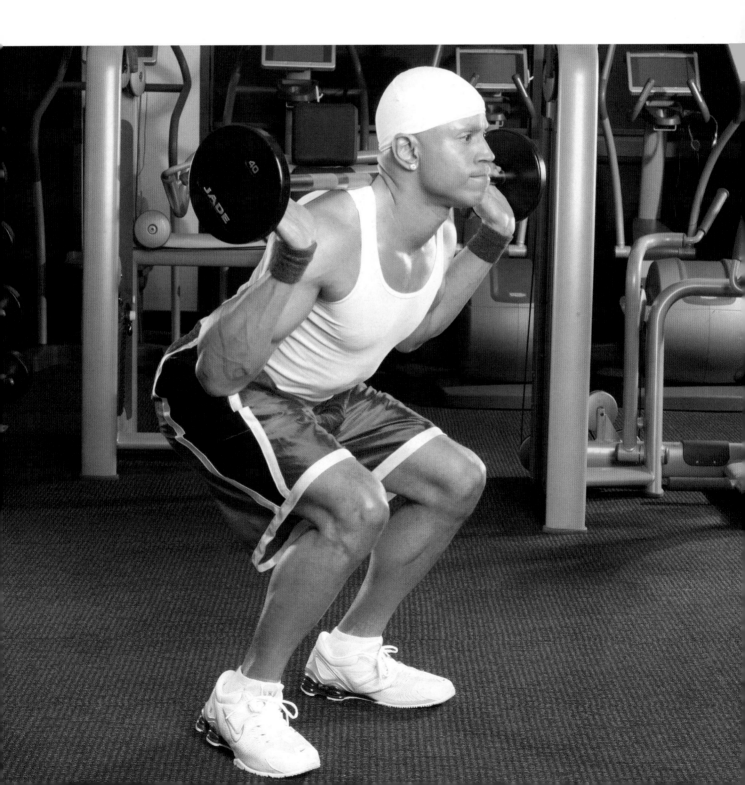

# Bent-Over Barbell Row

1. Hold a loaded barbell at arms' length and, keeping your back flat, lean forward so your torso is about 10 degrees short of being parallel with the floor. Use an overhand grip with your hands roughly shoulder-width apart. (Experiment. There is no one correct hand placing. This is a democracy—pick your own and go to work.) Bend your knees slightly to prevent lower-back strain during the lift. This is the start position.

2. Breathe deep and pull the bar up, exhaling as it approaches your navel. Don't swing the weight up; keep your body tight. Keep breathing throughout: no bonus points for underwater breathing techniques.

3. Lower the bar back to the start position without rounding your back.

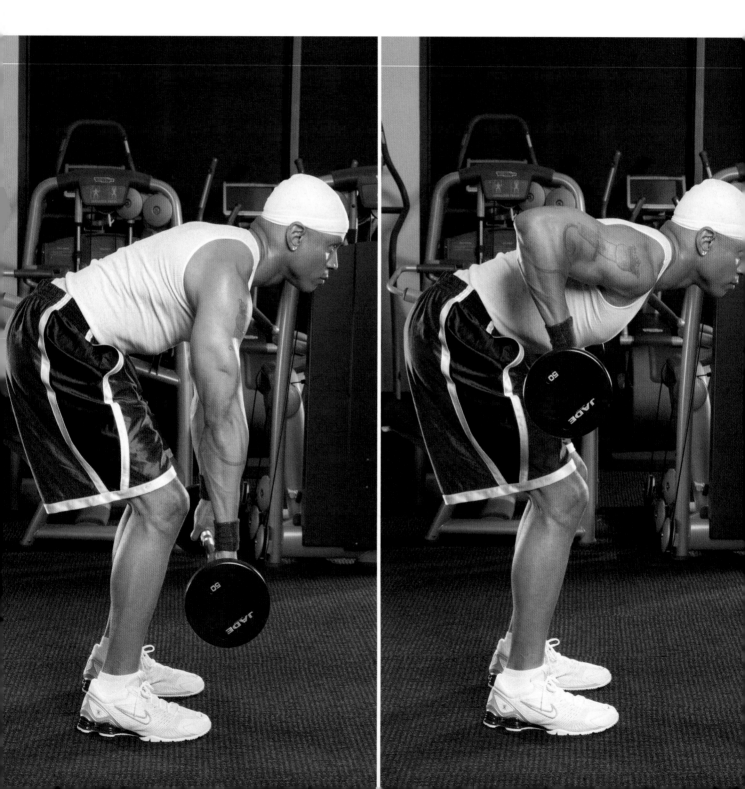

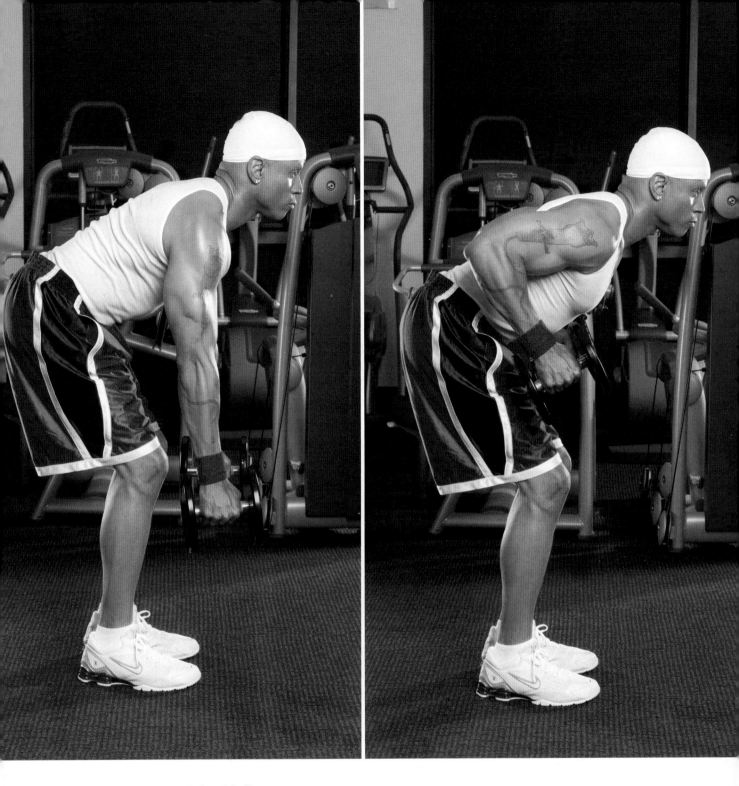

## Bent-Over Dumbbell Row

1. Hold dumbbells at arms' length and, keeping your back flat, lean forward so your torso is about 10 degrees short of being parallel with the floor. Bend your knees slightly to prevent lower-back strain during the lift. This is the start position.

2. Breathe deep and pull the weights up, exhaling as they approach your navel.

3. Lower the weights back to the start position without rounding your back.

# Bent-Over Lateral Raise

1. Stand with your feet planted on the floor, and lean forward until your chest is nearly horizontal.

2. Reach down and grab the weights already positioned at your feet. Use an overhand, thumbless grip. Let the dumbbells hang at arms' length, elbows bent slightly. This is the start position.

3. Raise both dumbbells in a circular motion until both arms are parallel with the floor, keeping your pinkies above your thumbs. Exhale during the ascent. Pause for a one- or two-count at the top.

4. Slowly lower both dumbbells back to the start position. Inhale during the descent.

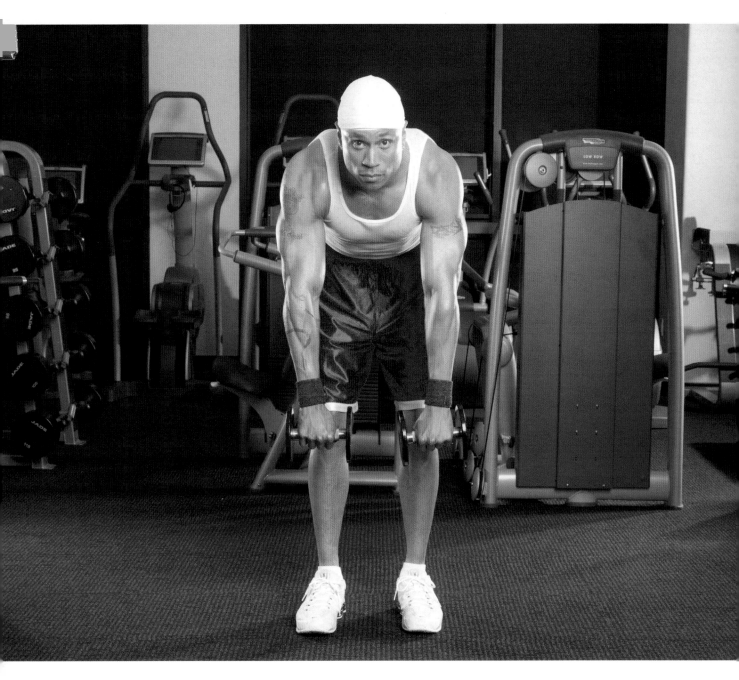

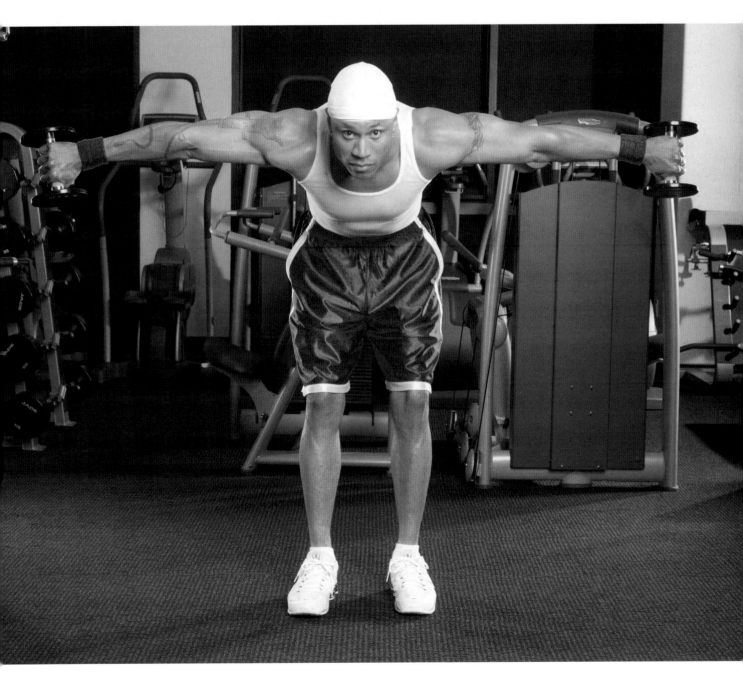

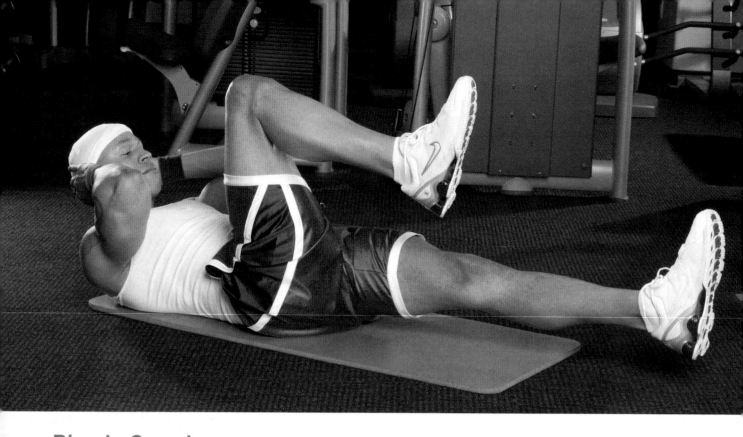

## Bicycle Crunch

1. Lie on your back with your hands behind your head.
2. Raise your legs 2 inches or so off the floor. This is the start position.
3. Draw your right knee toward you.
4. As you return it to the start position, simultaneously bring your left knee toward you.
5. Throughout, don't pull on your neck, don't let your feet touch the floor, and draw your navel down toward the floor.
6. The motion resembles pedaling a bike, only you're on your back.

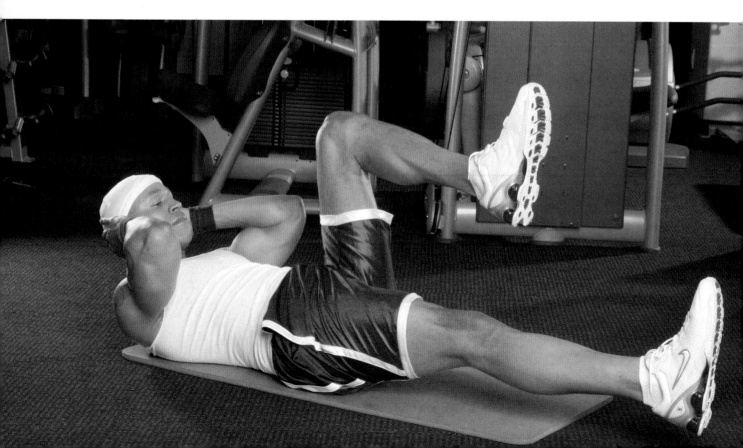

**Box Jump** 1. Stand in front of a sturdy box 15 to 30 inches high or several stacked aerobics steps.

2. Without swinging your arms, jump up as high as you can and land on the box. Exhale as you're jumping.

3. Try to land easy: Never land with your knees past the plane of your feet; never lower your hips past your knees when landing.

4. Return to the start position by stepping down.

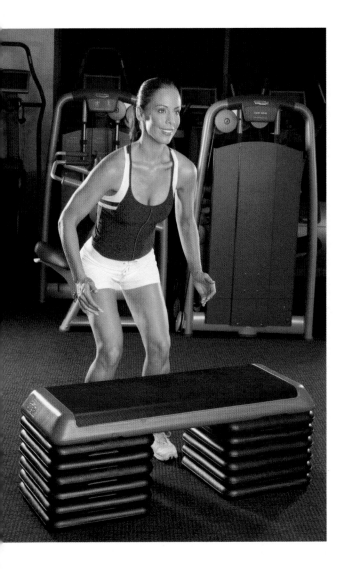

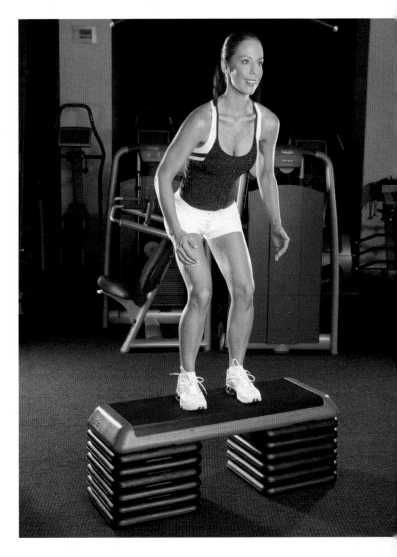

# Burpee with Jump

1. Stand in place with your arms at your sides, feet shoulder-width apart. This part of the exercise isn't hard for you—we're sure of that—so it's not pictured.

2. Squat down in a catcher's position and place your palms on the floor.

3. Without pausing, kick your legs back to assume a pushup position: back straight, gaze forward.

4. Do one pushup.

5. Reverse the movement to return to the catcher's position.

6. Return to the start position, but leave the floor in a squat jump.

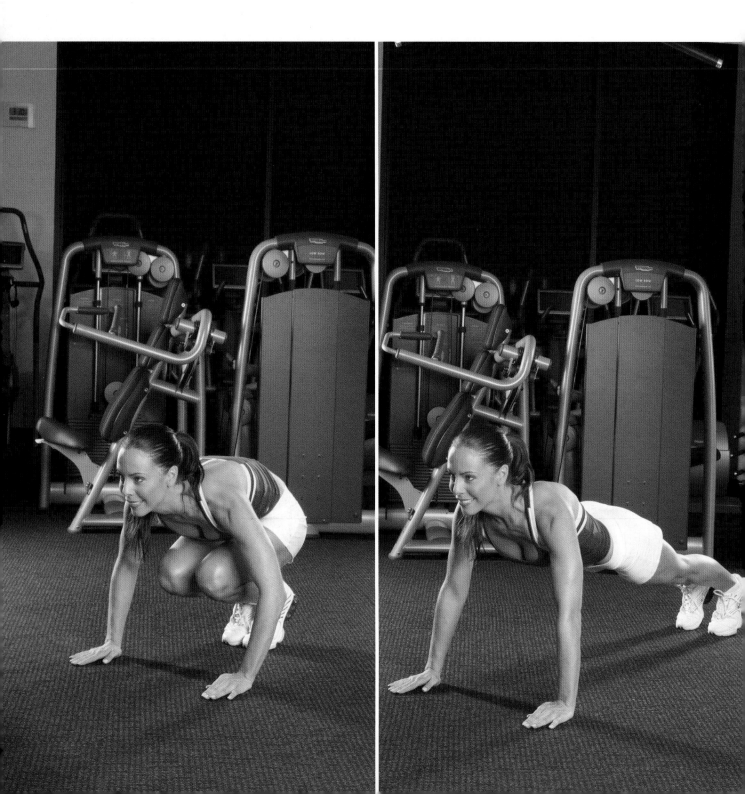

# **S**COOTER'S *MUSCLE-BUILDING TIP*

Slow down the speed of your repetitions until you really *feel* the muscles you're supposed to be working. Only then should you go faster.

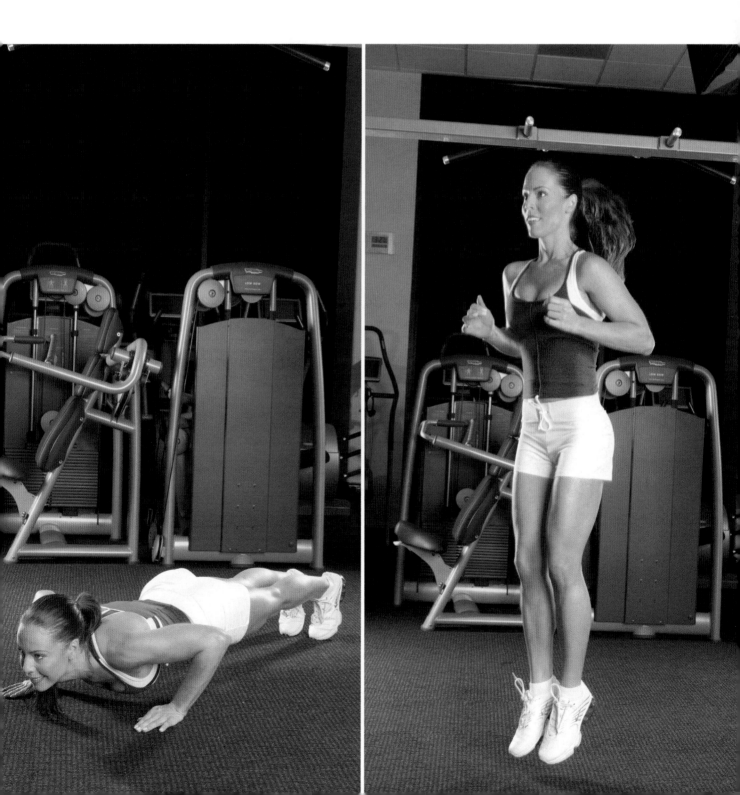

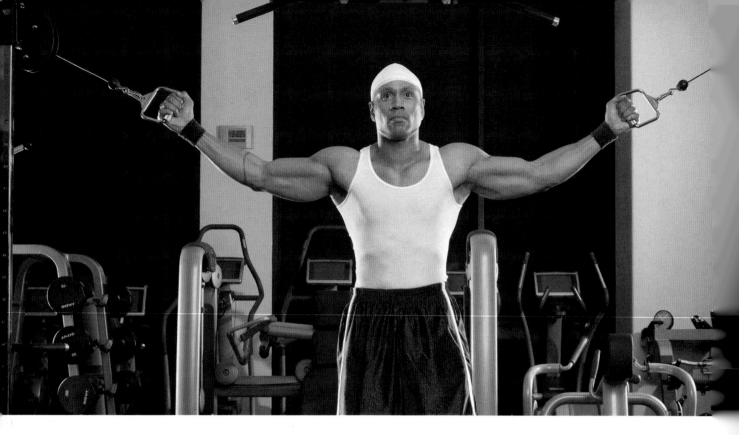

## Cable Crossover

1. Stand in between cable stacks, holding stirrup handles attached to high pulleys. Your gaze should be fixed forward.

2. Step forward about 18 inches.

3. Pull the handles in front of you in an arc, as if you're hugging a tree, until the handles meet at your lower abdomen. Your hands should actually cross.

4. Squeeze your pecs hard for a two-count and then return the handles to the start position.

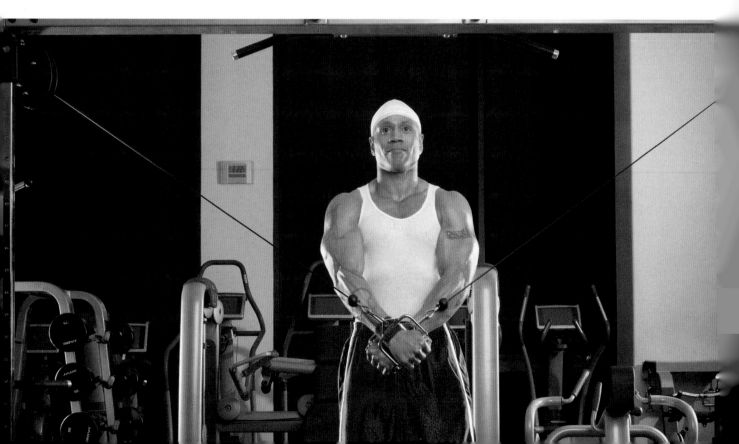

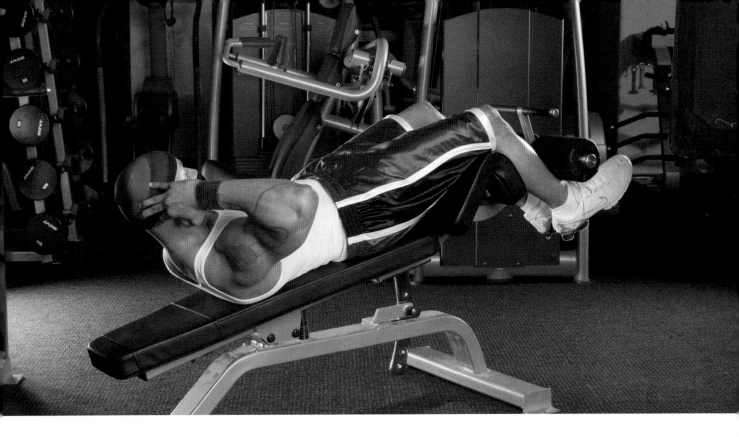

# Decline Situp

1. Lie on a decline situp bench and lock your feet under the rollers.

2. Place your hands over your ears, which will keep you from pulling on your neck as your body comes up. This is the start position.

3. Breathe deep as you start the movement by curling your lower abs while pushing your pelvis into the bench. Come up to where your elbows and knees meet, exhaling on the way up.

4. After your elbows meet your knees, slowly return to the start position. Inhale as you go.

5. Situps can also be done on an incline bench, where your head is above your feet, not below them; or on a flat bench or the floor, so that your head and feet begin in the same horizontal plane.

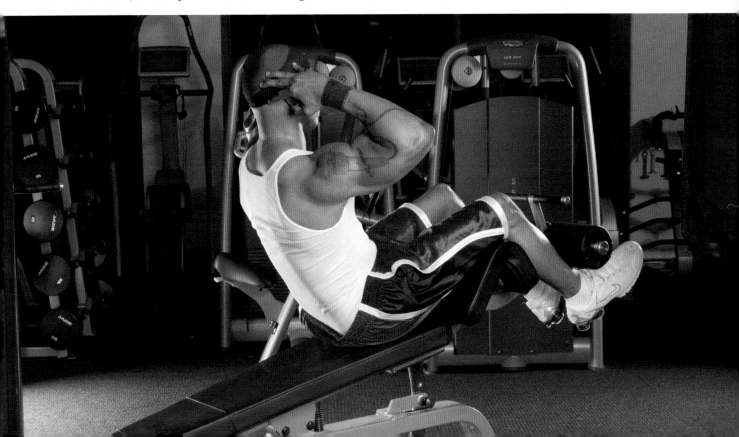

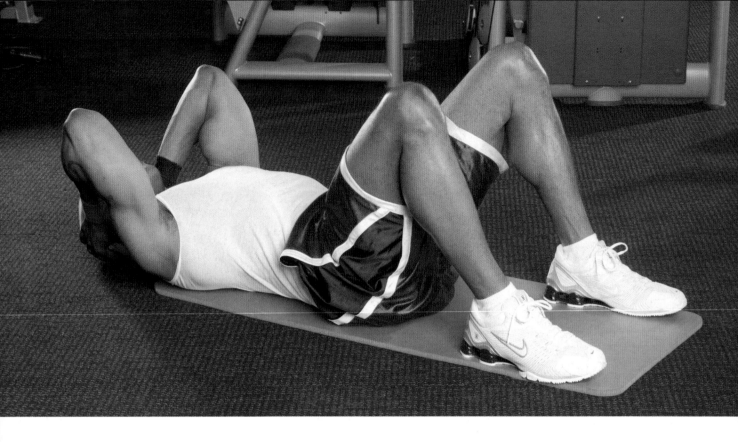

## Crunch

1. With this movement you will again be on your back—yo, stop thinking like that! Place your fingers at your temples as if you're trying to block out the instructions Scooter Pie is barking at you.

2. Bend your knees into upside-down Vs. This is the start position.

3. Contract your abs to bring your shoulders off the floor. At the same time you're crunching forward, press your lower back into the floor. Inhale during the ascent.

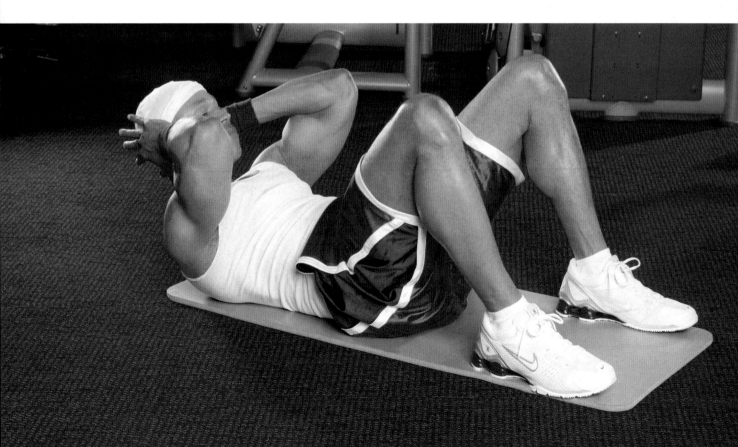

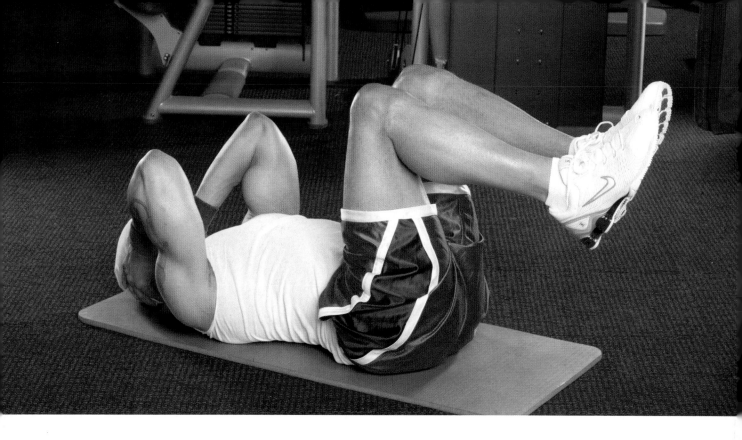

4. Return to the start, but don't let your shoulders touch the floor. Exhale on the descent.

5. To make the exercise more difficult, raise your feet off the floor and bend your knees so that your legs form Ls when viewed from the side, as shown in the photos above and below.

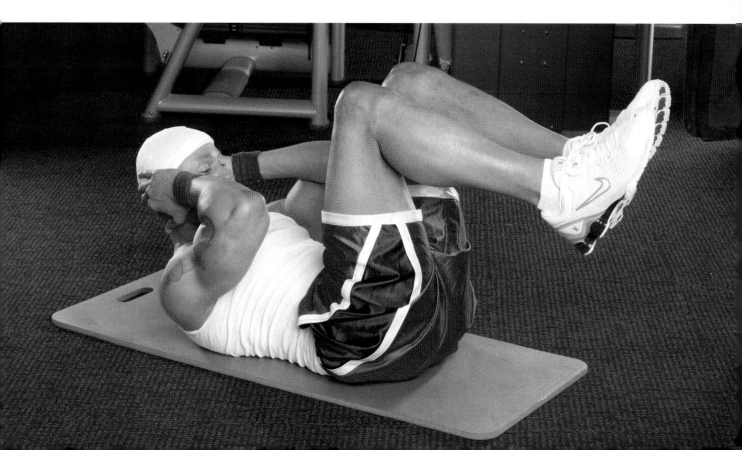

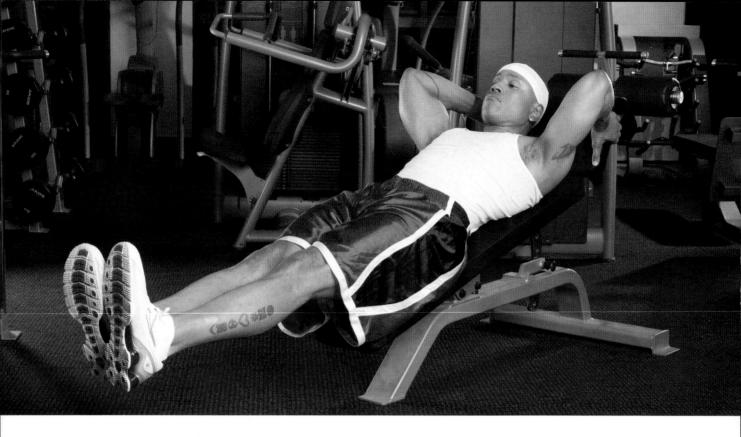

## Incline Knee-In/Hip Thrust

1. Sit on an incline bench so that your legs hang off it, and place your hands behind you for support. Extend your feet in front of you, feet together. This is the start position.

2. Draw your knees in toward your chest, and then raise your hips off the bench to thrust your legs toward the ceiling. Hold for a second or two.

3. Return to the intermediate position before returning to the start position.

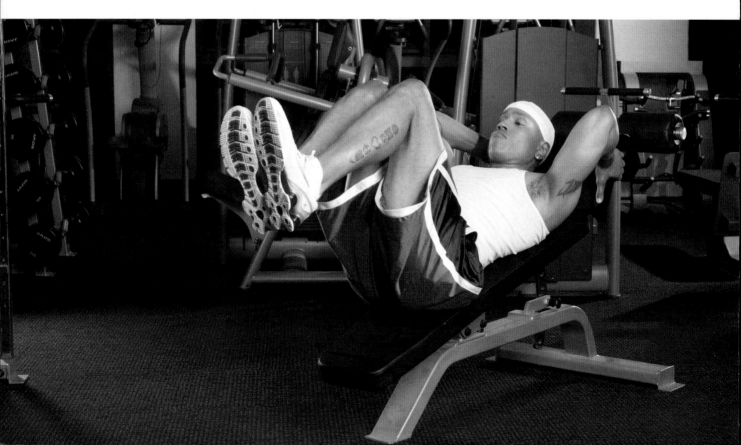

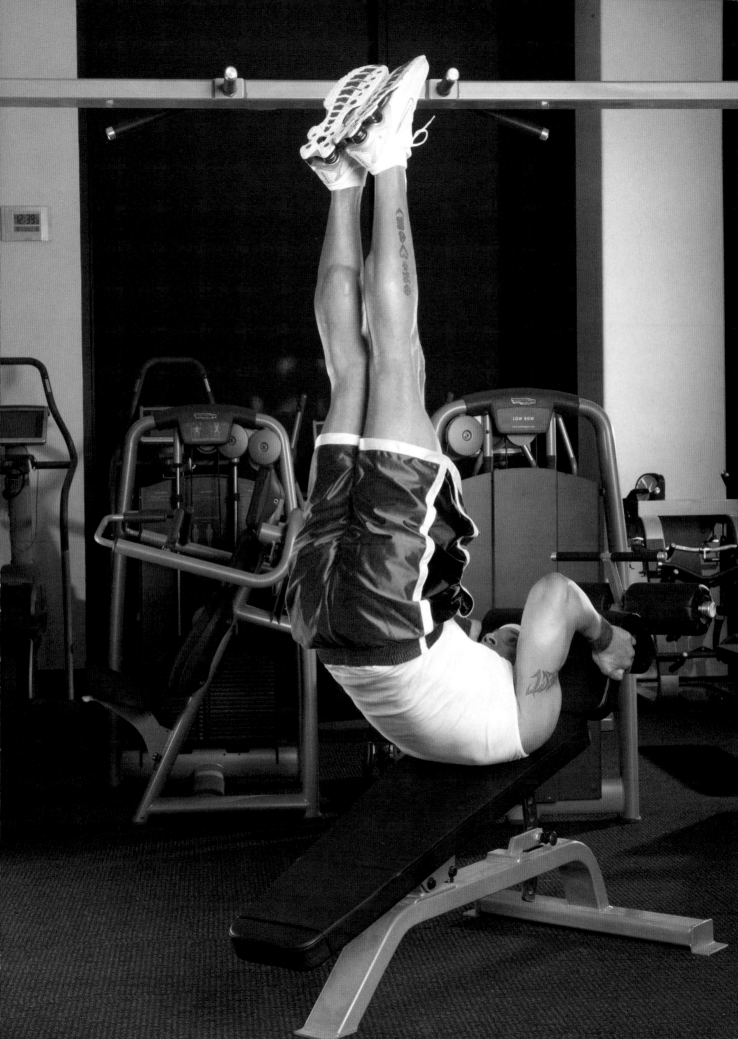

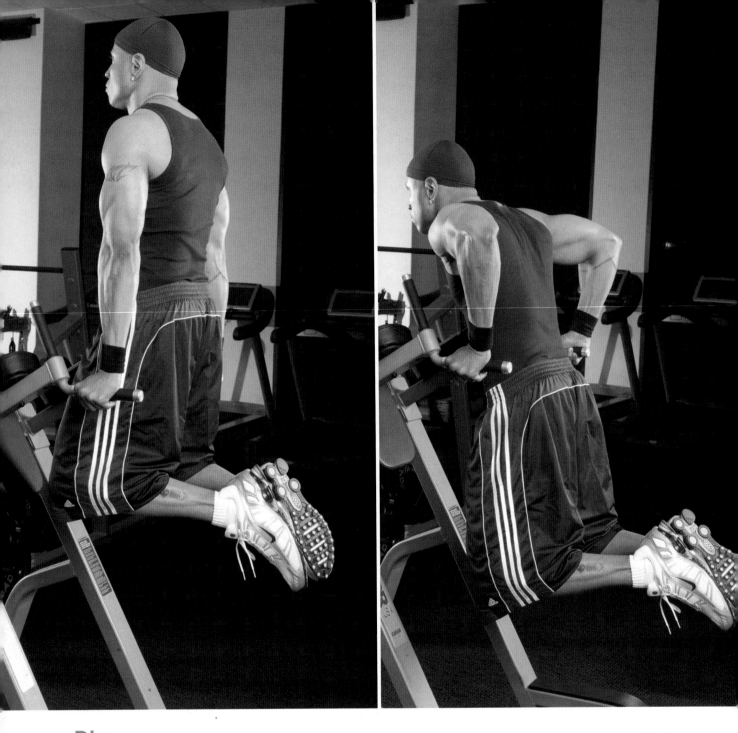

**Dip** 1. If the bars are parallel, don't worry about this, but if the bars are angled, select the narrow end, where your hands will be 10 to 12 inches apart. Once you've established your grip, push yourself up so that your arms are straight and your knees are bent 90 degrees, with your feet tucked behind you. This is the start position.

2. Without inclining your torso forward—which would shift the emphasis from your triceps to your pecs—bend your arms to lower your body until your elbows form 90-degree angles.

3. Inhale during a measured descent, about a three-count, controlling the rep at all times. Drop quickly and you risk damaging the delicate architecture of your shoulder joints.

4. From the bottom, straighten your elbows to return to the start position at a two-count pace, again making sure to keep your back straight.

5. Exhale as you approach the top, and don't lock out your elbows hard at full extension. And keep them tucked in close to your body for the entire set.

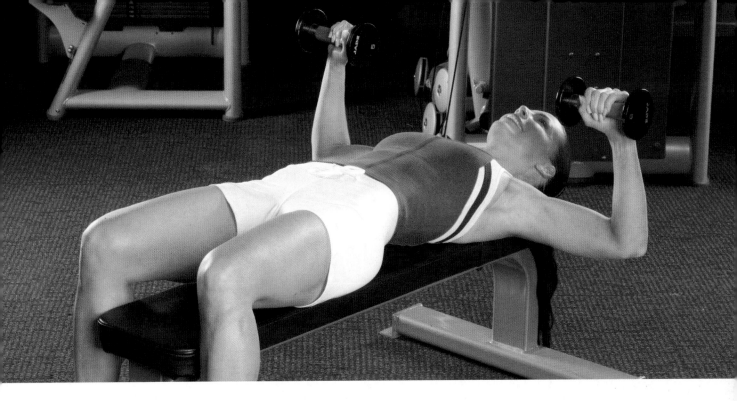

## Dumbbell Bench Press

1. Lie on a bench, holding dumbbells just outside your shoulders, palms facing forward, feet planted.

2. Squeeze your pecs to press the dumbbells up toward the ceiling in a slight arc and back about 10 degrees. Exhale deeply on the ascent.

3. Maintaining continuous tension on your chest muscles, bring the weights back to the start position, dropping your shoulders as the weights approach your body. Inhale on the descent.

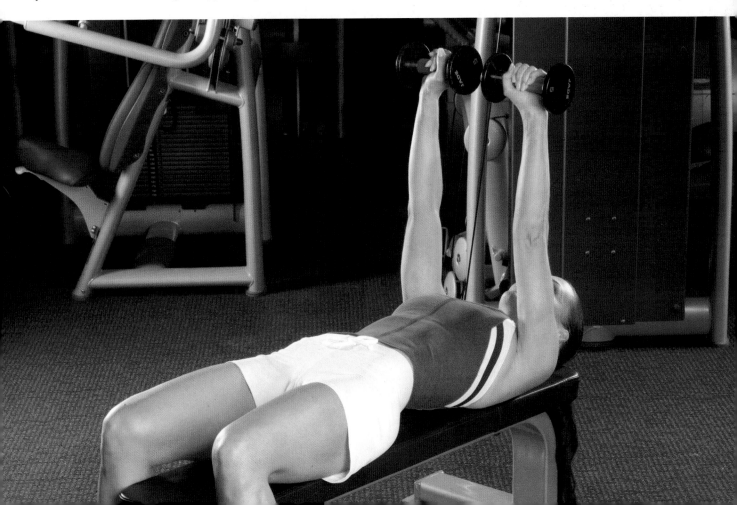

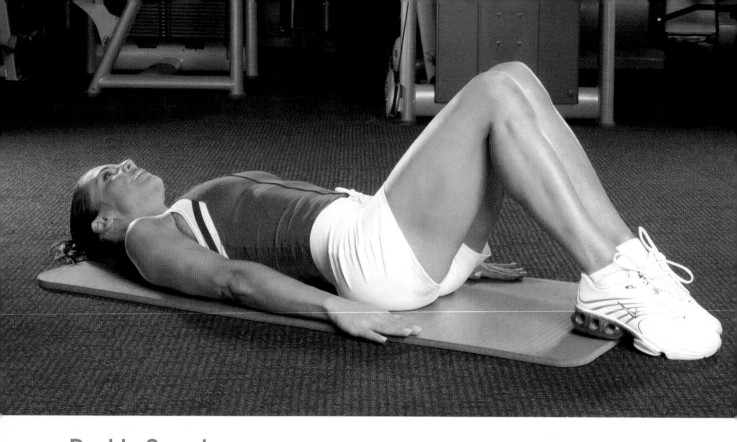

## Double Crunch

1. Lie on your back with your arms straight and beside your torso.

2. Bend your knees into upside-down Vs. This is the start position.

3. Contract your abs to bring your shoulders off the floor. As you crunch forward, bring your knees toward your elbows. The two halves of your body will come together like the accordion Scooter's brother played like a madman at his bar mitzvah.

4. Return to the start, but don't let your shoulders touch the floor. Exhale on the descent.

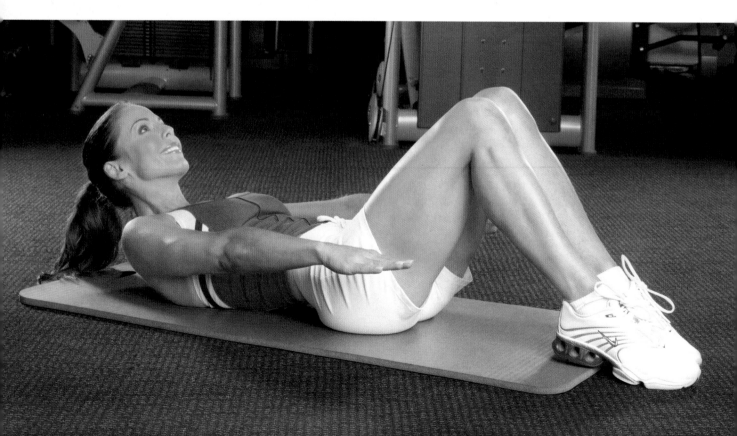

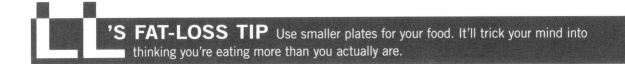
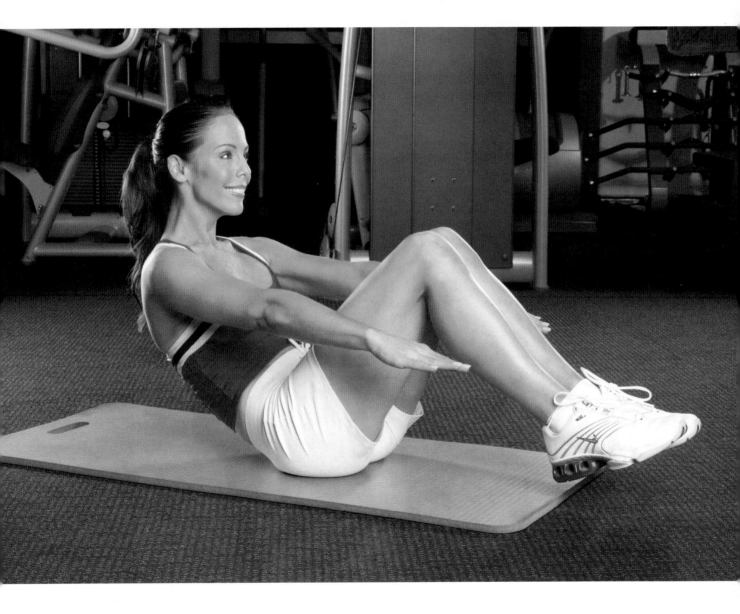

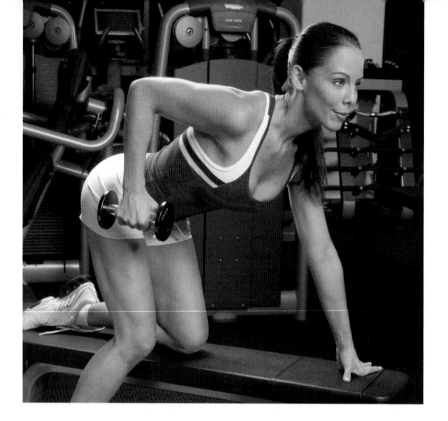

## Dumbbell Kickback

1. Holding a dumbbell in one hand, place the opposite knee on a flat bench and bend at the waist until your back is nearly parallel with the floor.

2. Bend your elbow so the dumbbell faces your outer thigh and your elbow points back. This is the start position.

3. Extend your working arm straight back behind your body, exhaling as you go, until your elbow locks. (Don't jerk the dumbbell, though, or you'll injure yourself.) At full extension your arm should be parallel with the floor.

4. Contract the triceps for a two-count and then return slowly to the start position, inhaling as you go.

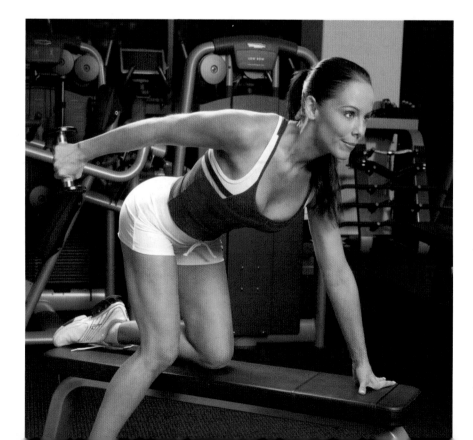

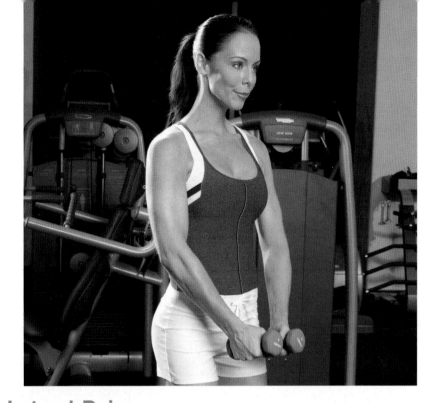

## Dumbbell Lateral Raise

1. Okay, if you're tired, you can sit down and relax. We kid! It's harder to sit than it is to keep moving, so let's get to work. Hold dumbbells in front of you at arms' length, except for a slight bend at the elbows, so that your palms face each other. This is the start position.

2. Pulling with your elbows, raise the dumbbells out in an arc so that your palms are facing down as the weights approach shoulder level. (I like going high because it requires more control than a lower finishing point, while placing a little more emphasis on the middle heads of the deltoids.) At the top, count to two.

3. Return to the start position, stopping 1 inch or so before your quads. Never relax in the bottom position by allowing the weights to rest against your outer thighs, not even for a second. The goal is to keep tension on the target muscles continuously for the duration of your set. Do these right and you'll feel your shoulders burning and the fire engines coming—only they won't be able to put out the fire.

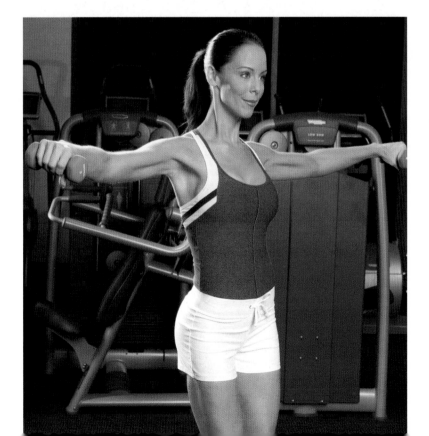

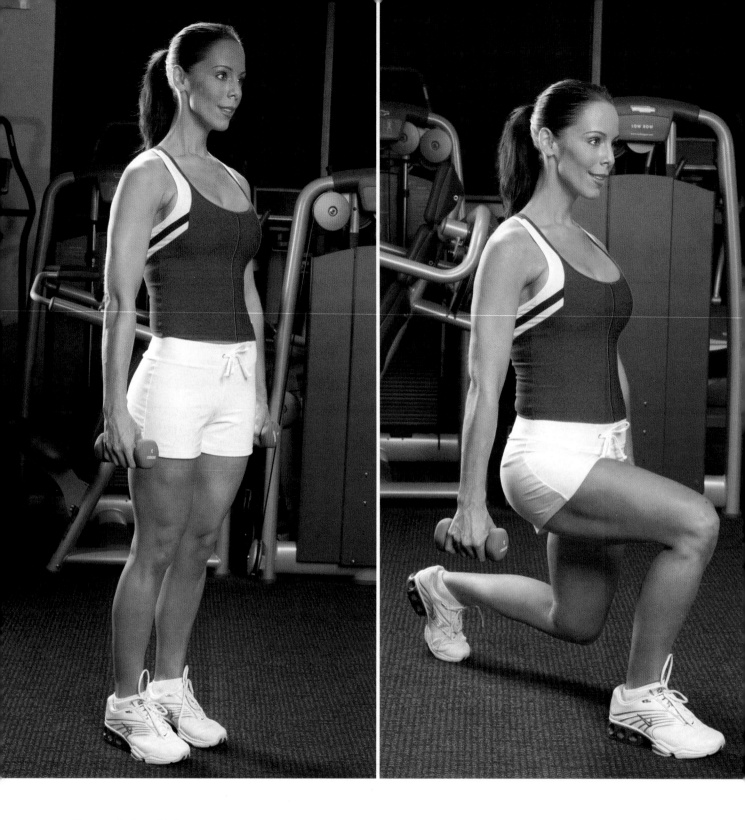

# Dumbbell Lunge

1. Grab a pair of matching dumbbells from the rack.

2. Hold them at arms' length at your sides, so your thumbs face forward.

3. Step forward with either leg and bend that lead knee, descending with your torso remaining erect. As you step forward, allow your trailing leg to bend until your back knee almost touches the ground.

4. Return to the start position.

5. Repeat using the other leg. Continue alternating for the duration of the set.

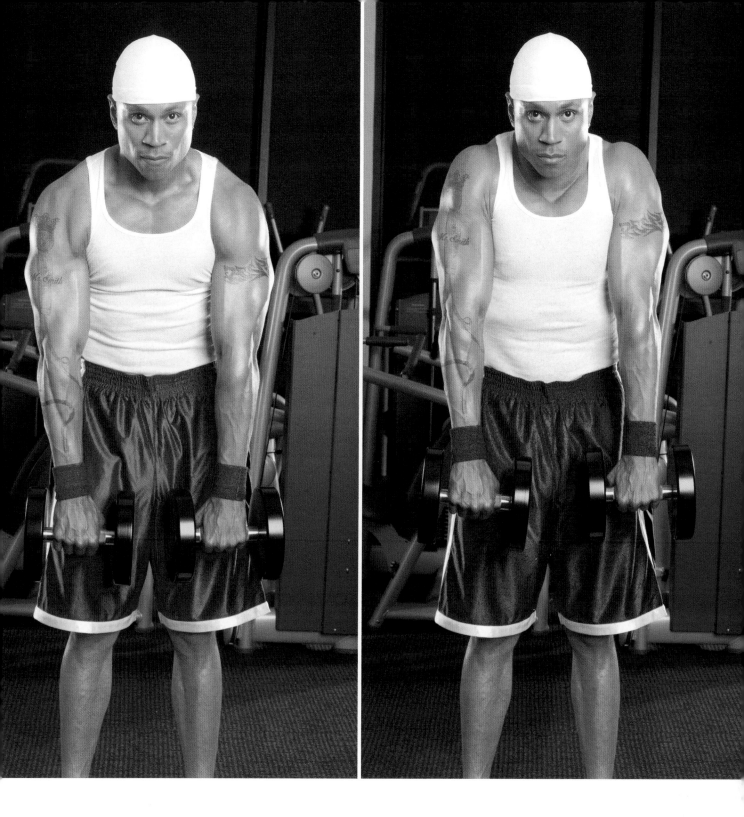

# Dumbbell Shrug
1. Hold a pair of dumbbells at your sides so your palms face your quads.

2. Tilt your shoulders down 10 degrees. This is the start position.

3. Exhale as you raise your shoulders straight up, trying to touch your ears.

4. Hold for a two-count and return to the start position.

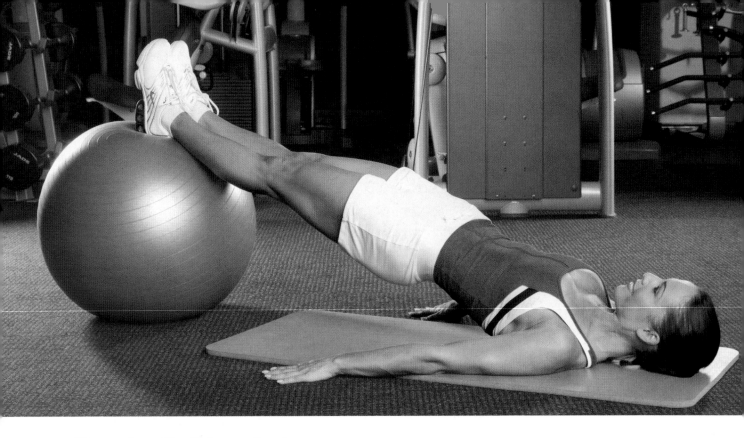

## Exercise Ball Leg Curl

1. Lie on the floor faceup with your ankles resting on top of an exercise ball. Your arms should be extended for balance.

2. Raise your hips off the round until your body forms a straight diagonal. Only your head and shoulder blades should be touching the floor or mat. This is the start position.

3. Keeping your body in this position, bend your knees and draw in your ankles to roll the ball as far as you can toward you. Your heels should approach your butt.

4. Roll the ball back to the start position.

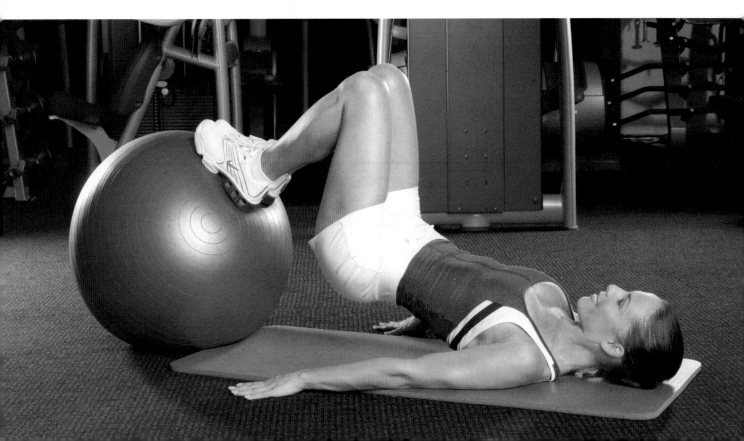

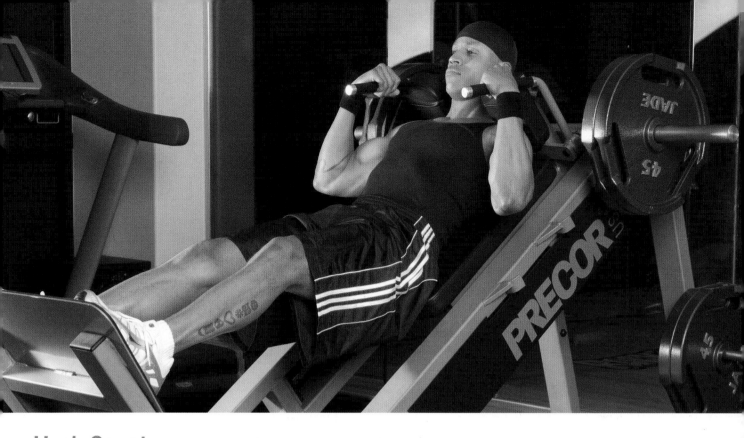

## Hack Squat

1. Stand in the machine so your back is flat against the sled's pad. Position yourself so that your shoulders fit snugly up and under the pads. Your feet should be planted shoulder-width apart.

2. Grasp the handles and release the locks. This is the start position.

3. Take a deep breath and descend until your thighs are parallel with the floor.

4. Exhale as you push through your heels to return to the start position, stopping just short of where your knees lock out. You don't want to jam your knee joints.

5. Make sure your back stays flat against the pad throughout the entire set.

6. Don't let your knees travel out past the plane of your feet.

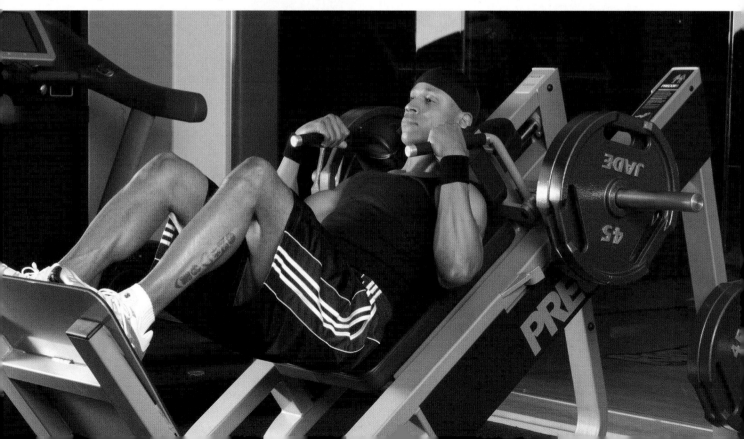

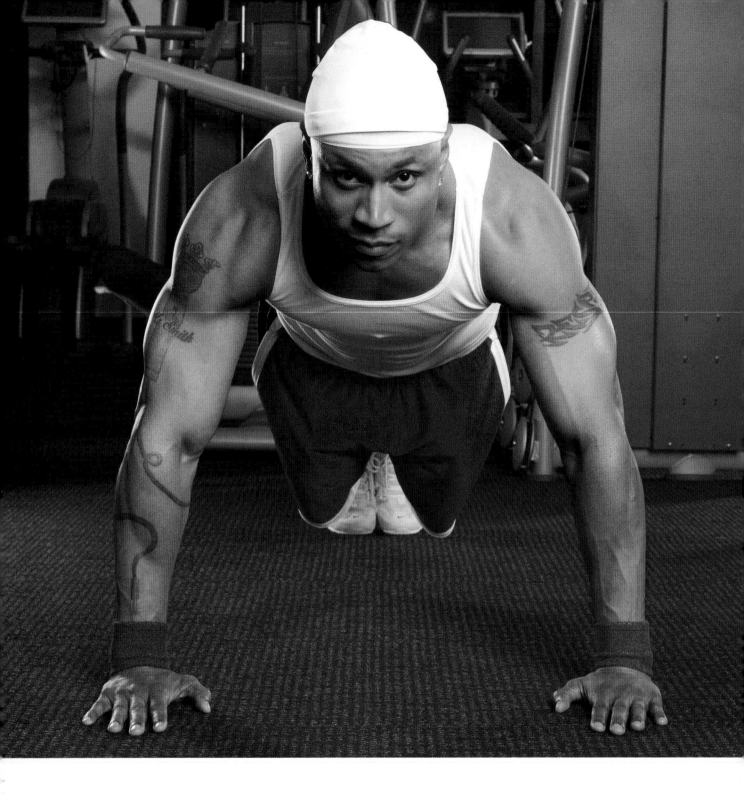

**Explosive Pushup** 1. Begin in your regular pushup position: body in alignment, arms extended, abs tight. This is the start position.

2. Bend your elbows to lower your body until it is only an inch or so off the ground.

3. Instead of returning to the start position normally, "explode" your body back up—imagine trying to push your hands through the floor—with the goal being to get your hands and torso to leave the floor momentarily.

4. Once you've mastered this version, try getting your hands, torso, and feet off the floor, as shown bottom right. Go airborne.

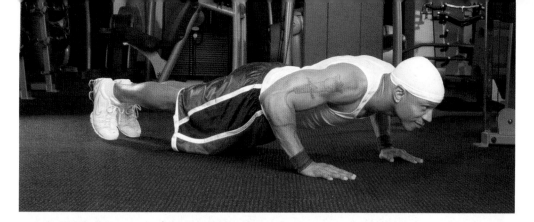

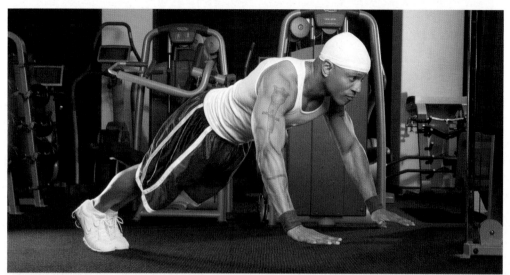

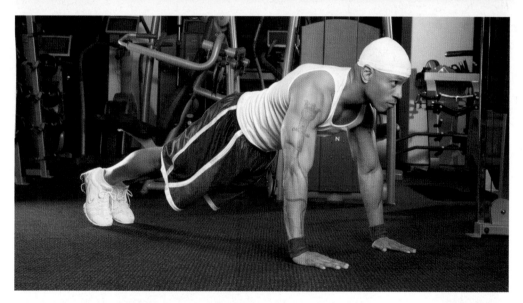

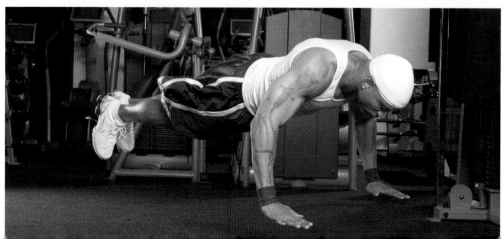

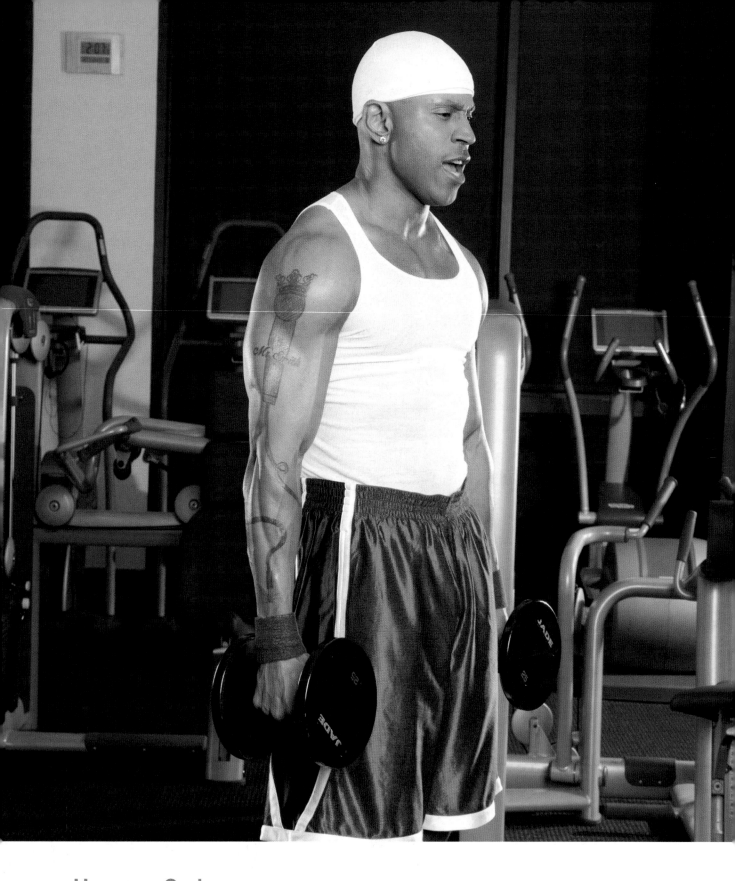

## Hammer Curl
1. Stand holding dumbbells at your sides at arms' length, with your palms facing each other so that your thumbs aim forward.

2. Keeping your elbows fixed at your sides, lift the weights as high as you can toward your shoulders.

3. After pausing for a one-count, return the weights to the start position.

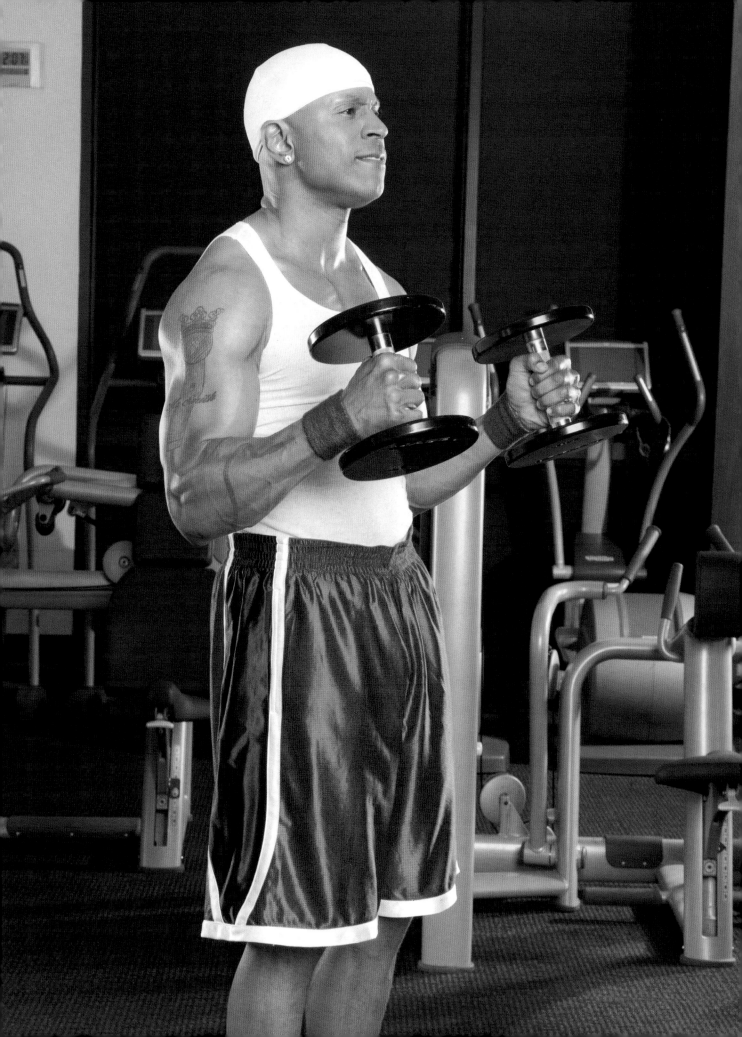

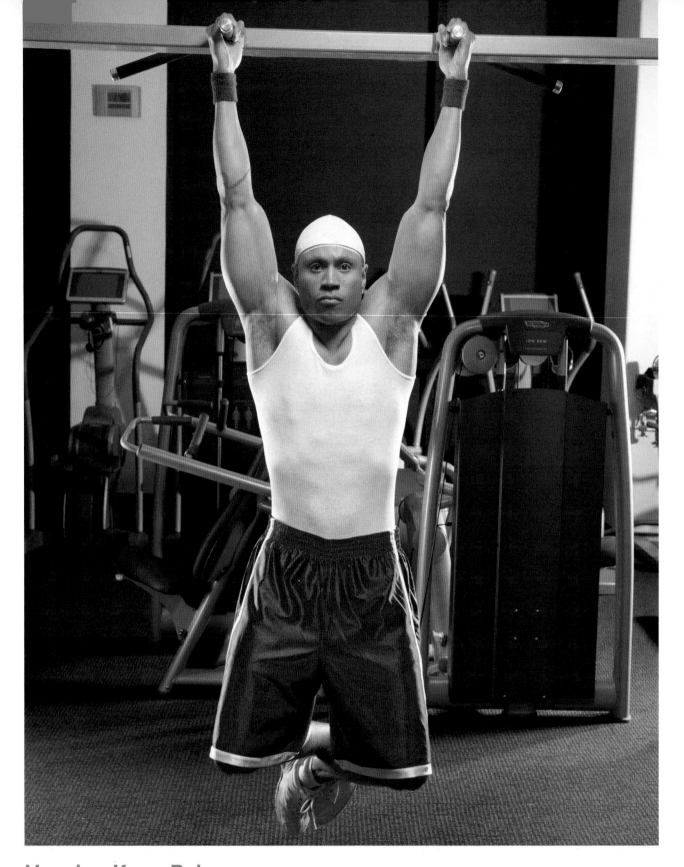

## Hanging Knee Raise

1. Either hang from a chinning bar or position yourself on a knee-raise apparatus with your forearms flush against the arm pads.

2. Hang with your knees bent and your legs free-floating. This is the start position.

3. Raise your knees up to the level of your midsection, really flexing your abs; don't swing. Exhale during the ascent.

4. Slowly and under control, lower your legs back to the start position. Exhale during the descent.

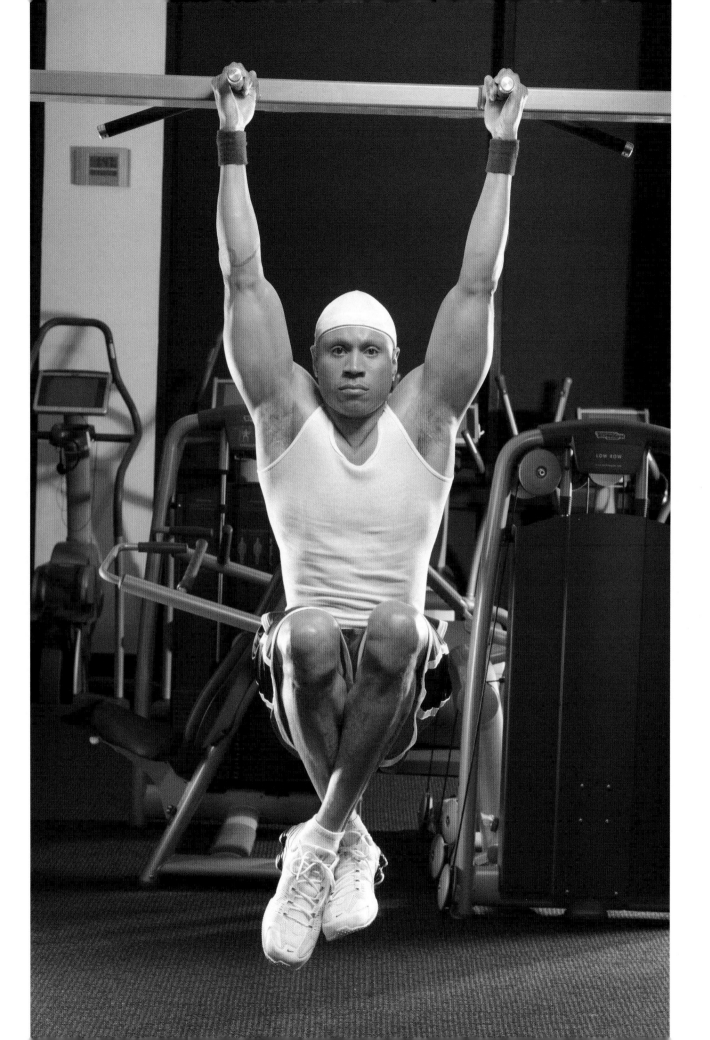

# Hanging Running Man

1. Grasp the handles of any two parallel bars in the gym. (Dipping bars are excellent for this movement.)

2. Assume an upright position by extending your arms and locking out your elbows. Raise one knee toward your chest, as if you're beginning to run.

3. As you lower it, raise the opposing knee as if you're pedaling a bike. But don't ride out of the gym.

4. If you're feeling masochistic, try doing dips *while* you're pedaling.

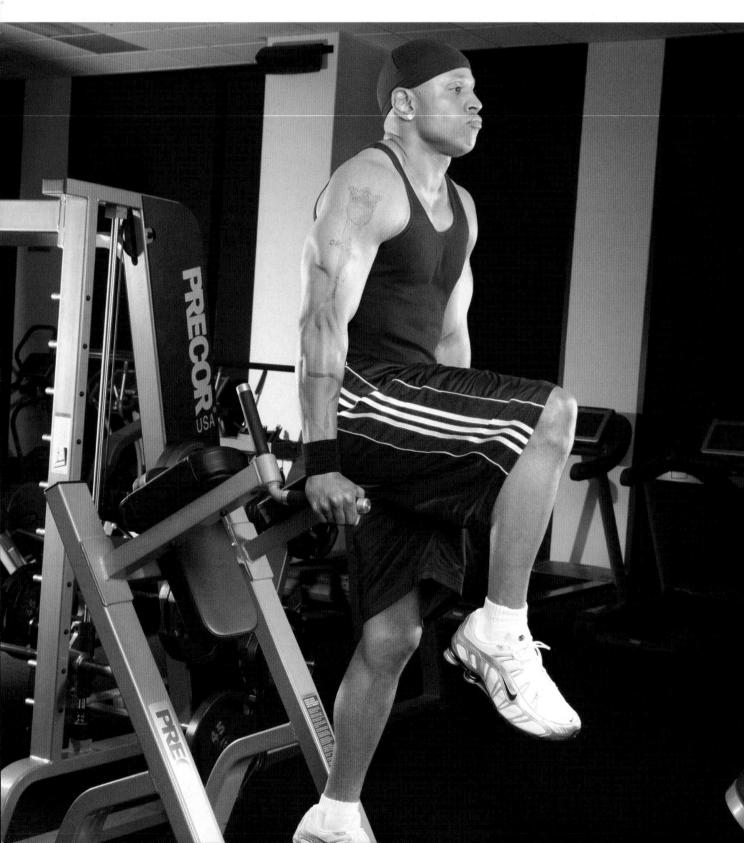

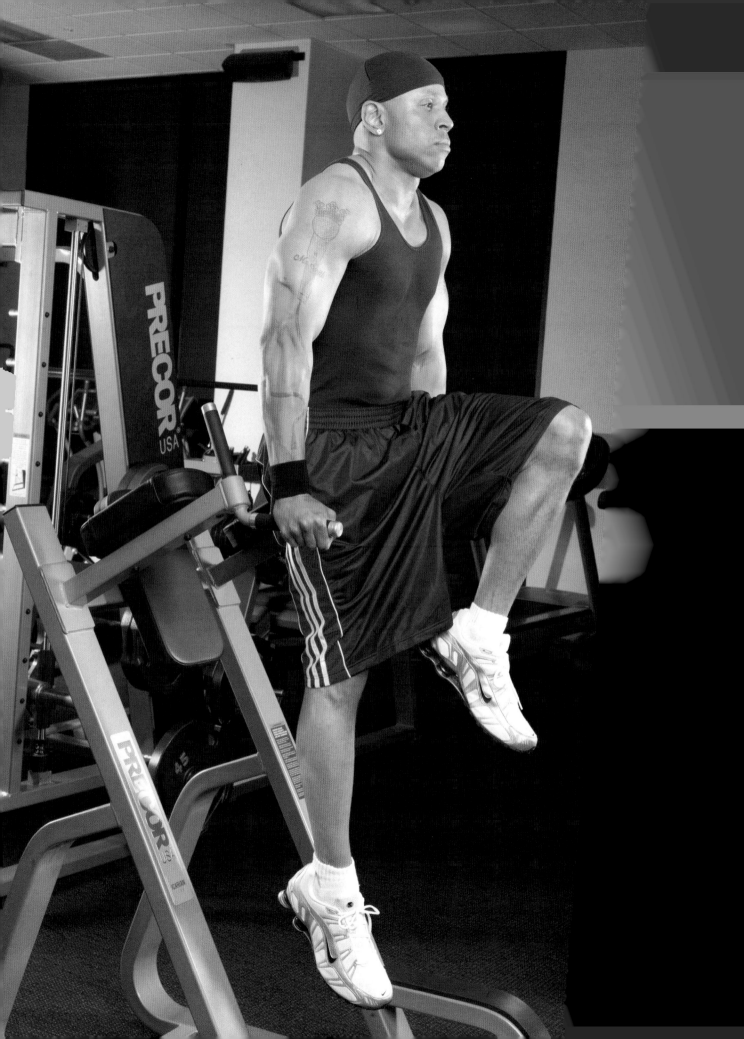

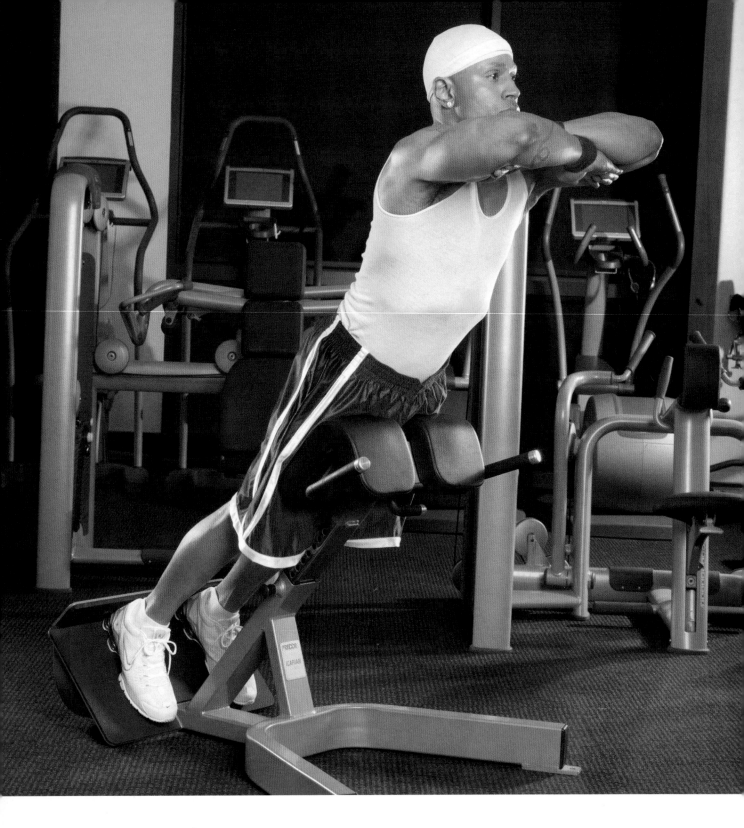

# Hyperextension

1. Lie facedown on the apparatus so that your ankles rest against the footpads and your torso floats freely over the end. Place your hands behind your head or across your chest.

2. Bend at the waist and lower your torso in a controlled manner, exhaling and keeping your back flat.

3. Reverse the movement to return to the start position, where your upper body is diagonal to the floor.

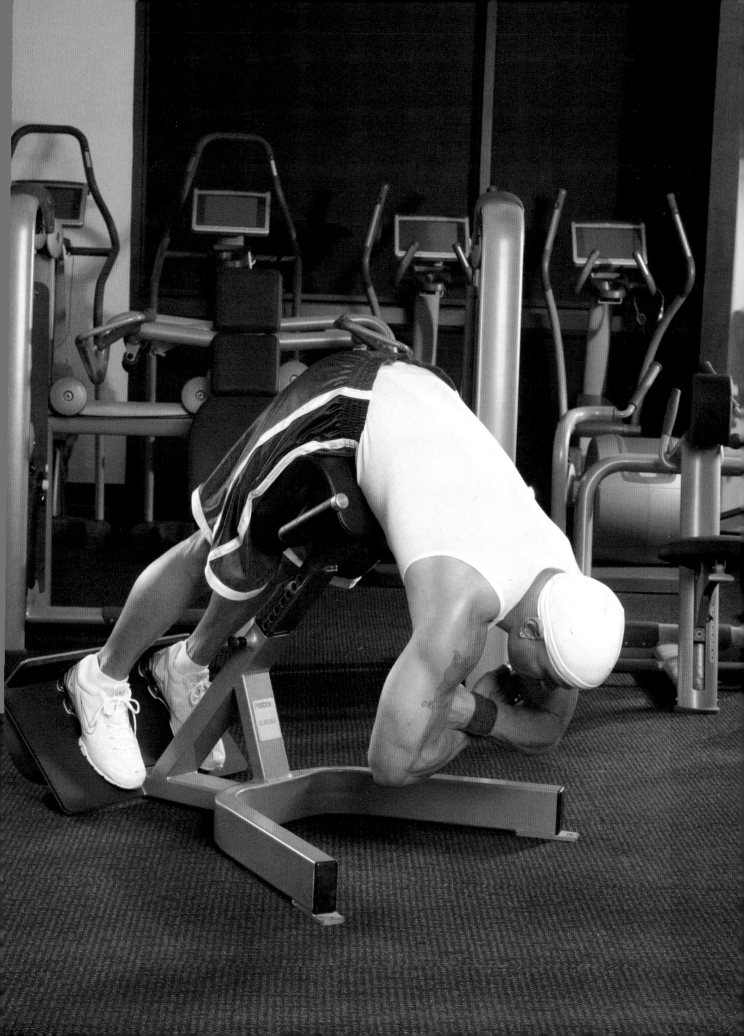

**Incline Barbell Bench Press (not pictured)** 1. Lie faceup with your back flat against the pad and your feet planted on the floor. The bench should be positioned as shown on the incline dumbbell bench press on the opposite page.

2. Unrack the bar and raise it above you at arms' length. This is the start position.

3. Lower the bar at a three-count until it touches your upper chest. Inhale during the descent.

4. Without "bouncing" off the bottom, push the weight back up at a two-count to the start position. Exhale during the ascent, and don't lock out your arms at the top.

5. Make sure your glutes remain on the bench, your eyes stay trained on the ceiling, and your wrists stay straight at all times.

When I think about the things we did
And I think about **you having my kids**
And I think about us sharing a crib
Losin' all that, God forbid
You deserve **flowers and candy,
the simple things**
In addition to the SL's, bigets and rings

—LL Cool J, **"Luv U Better," 2002**

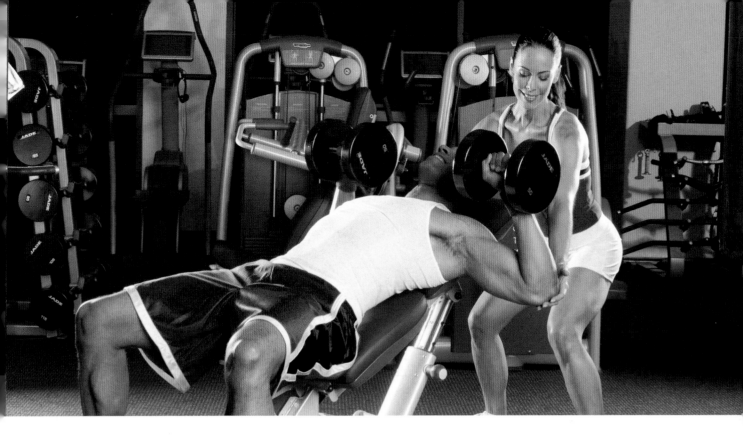

## Incline Dumbbell Bench Press
1. Lie on an incline bench holding dumbbells just outside your shoulders, palms facing up, feet planted.

2. Squeeze your pecs to press the dumbbells up toward the sky in a slight arc and back about 10 degrees. Exhale deeply on the ascent.

3. Bring the weights back to the start position. Inhale on the descent.

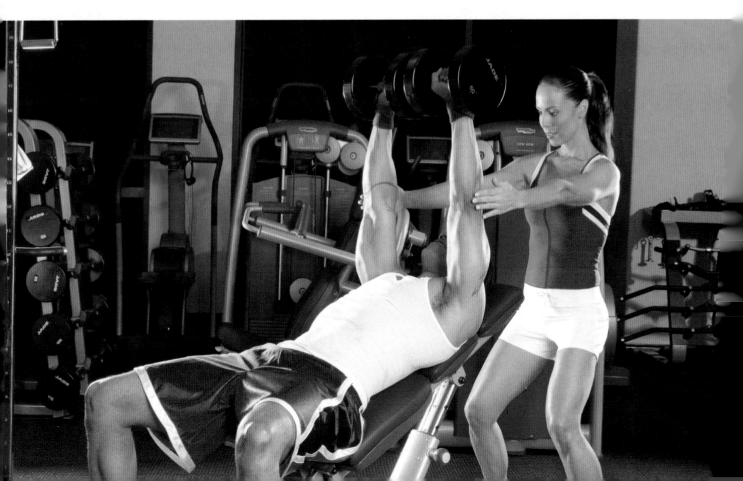

# Incline Dumbbell Curl

1. Set the incline bench at 60 degrees.

2. Lie back on the bench, holding a pair of dumbbells at arms' length so your palms face forward. Spread your stance for balance. This is the start position.

3. Curl the weights up to the front of your shoulders, exhaling as you keep your elbows down and back and in line with your shoulders. Squeeze!

4. Without rocking your body, inhale as you return the weights to the arms-extended position.

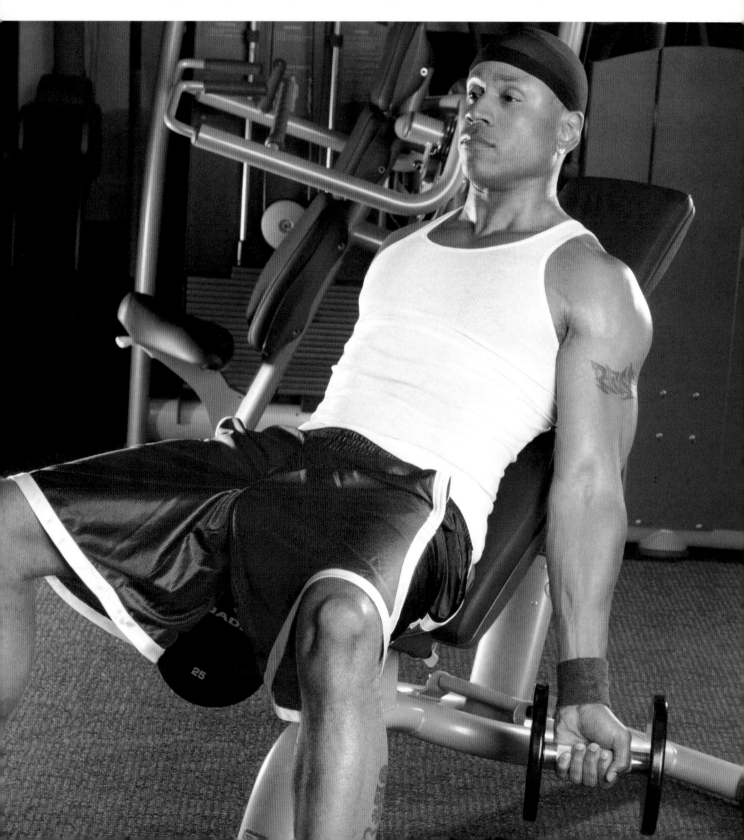

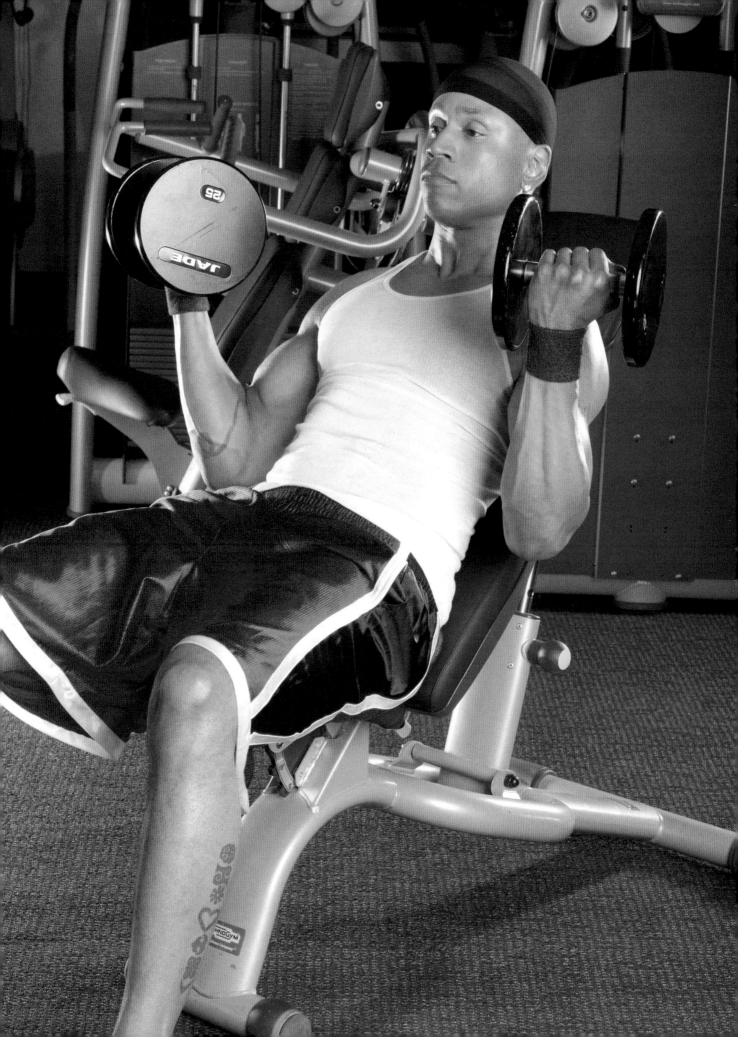

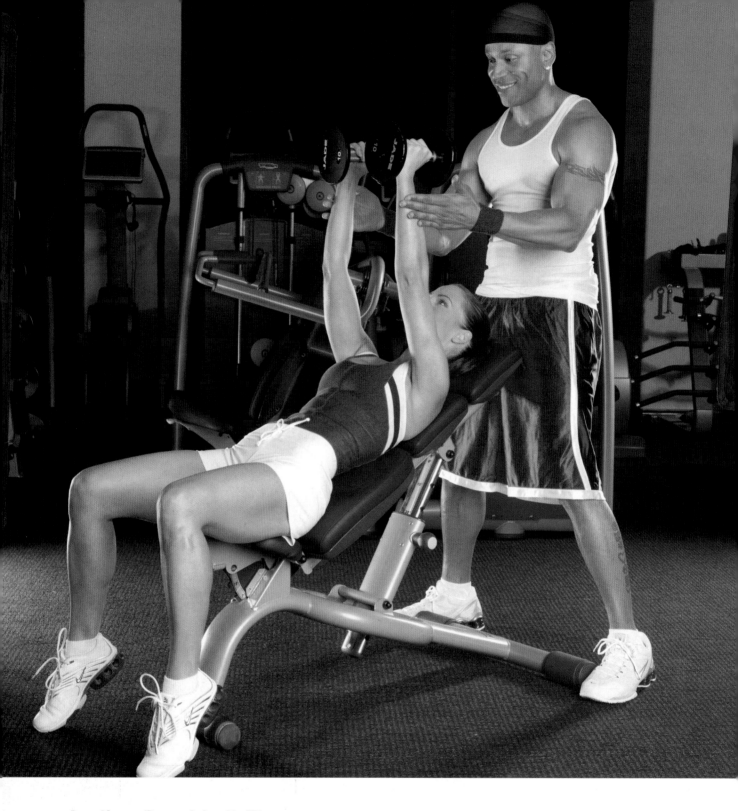

## Incline Dumbbell Fly
1. Holding dumbbells, lie back on a bench and plant your feet.

2. Raise the dumbbells to arms' length above you, palms facing each other, and bend your elbows very slightly. This is the start position.

3. In a controlled manner, lower the dumbbells in a semicircle until your elbows are outside of your armpits. Inhale deeply during the descent.

4. Stop for a slight pause at the bottom and then retrace the arc back to the start position. Exhale during the ascent.

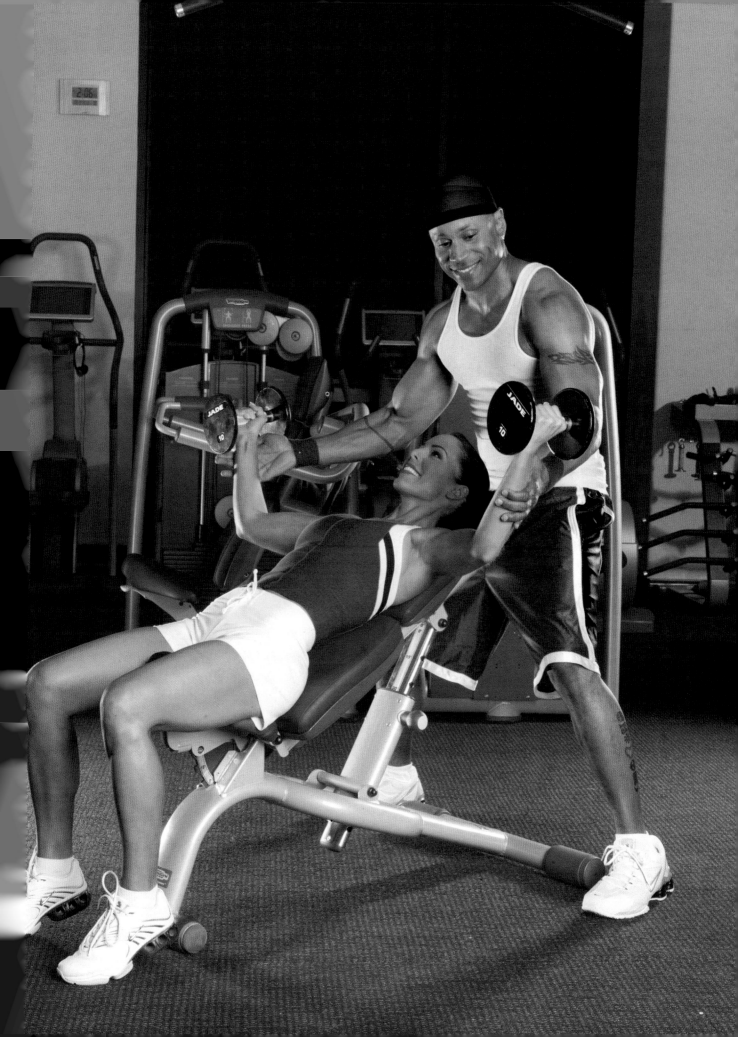

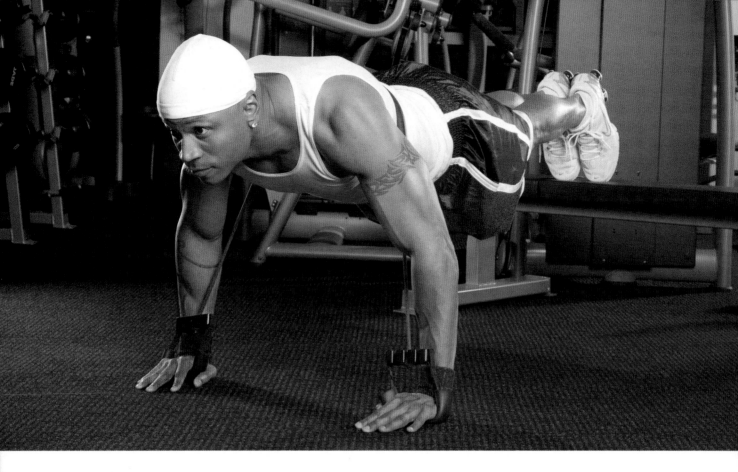

## Incline Pushup with Tubing

1. Assume the normal pushup position, arms extended. Only for this exercise, your feet should be elevated on a box or bench 12 to 15 inches high, and you should have rubber tubing wrapped around your back, with a handle in each hand.

2. Bend your elbows to lower your body to the floor.

3. Push to raise your torso back up. The tubing should make this half of the rep much harder than normal, especially as you approach the top.

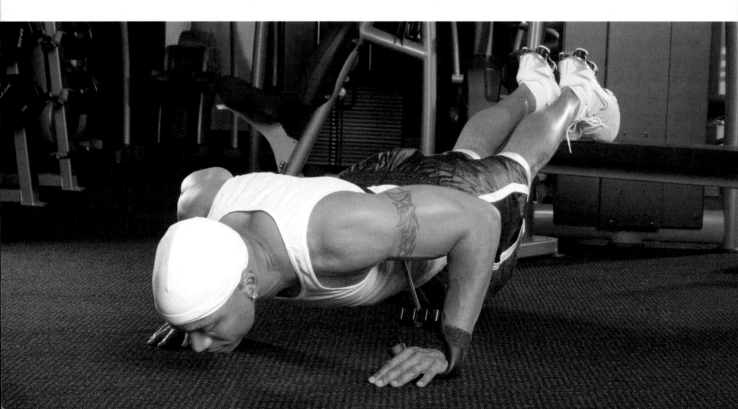

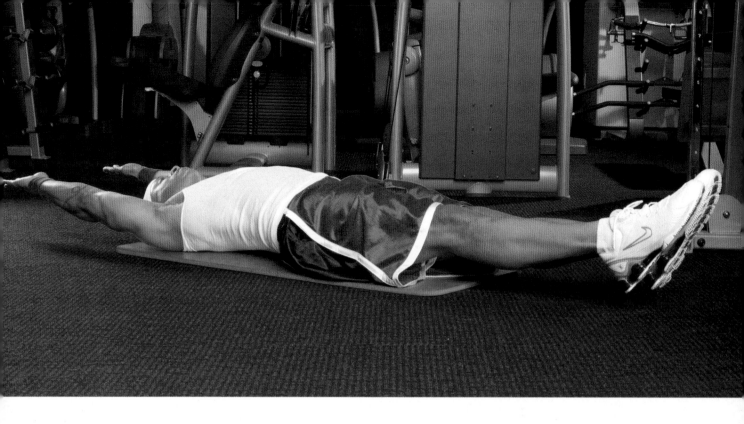

**Jackknife** 1. Lie on the floor with your arms extended behind your head and your legs extended in front of you. This is the start position.

2. Keeping your arms and legs straight, simultaneously lift all four limbs, trying to touch your toes with your hands—at which point you'll resemble a jackknife. Exhale in this top position.

3. Inhale as you return to the start position, only don't allow your feet to touch the ground. Leave about an inch of space between your feet and floor before starting the next rep.

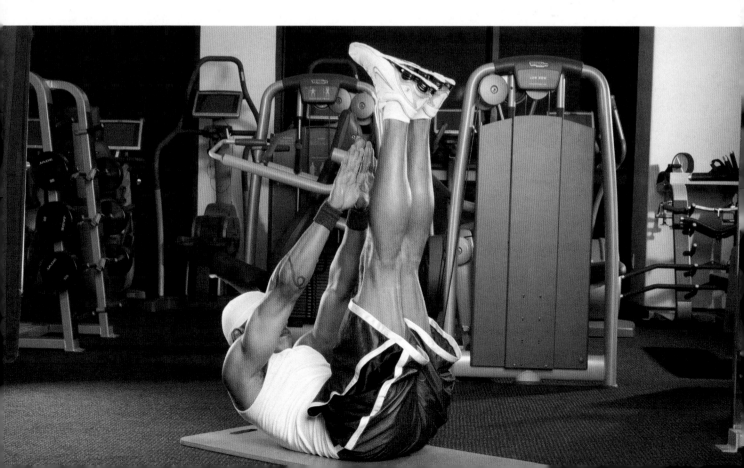

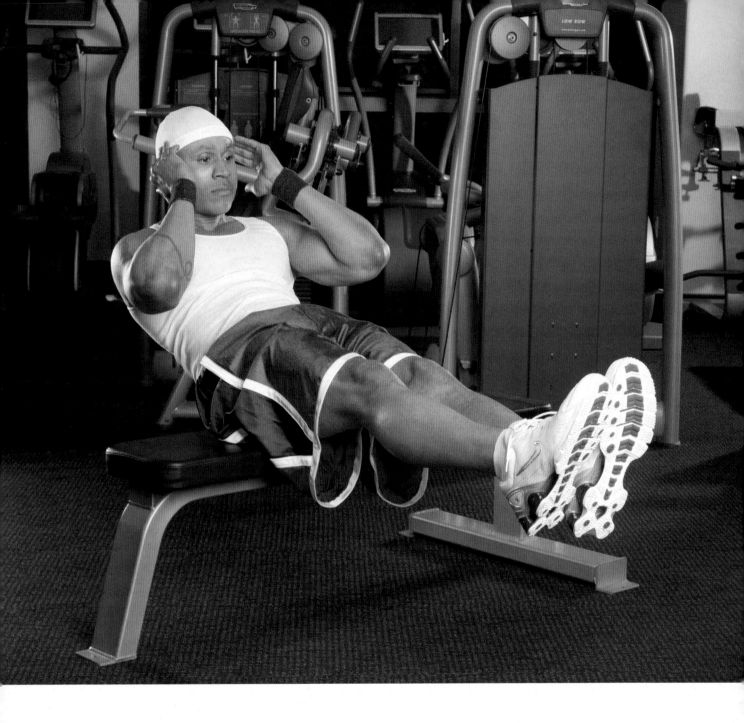

**Knee-In** 1. Sit perpendicular on a flat bench and place your hands at your temples. Extend your legs in front of you, feet together, your knees bent slightly.

2. Lean back. This is the start position.

3. Draw your knees in toward your chest while crunching your torso forward, until they meet, exhaling as you do this accordion-like move.

4. Return to the start position.

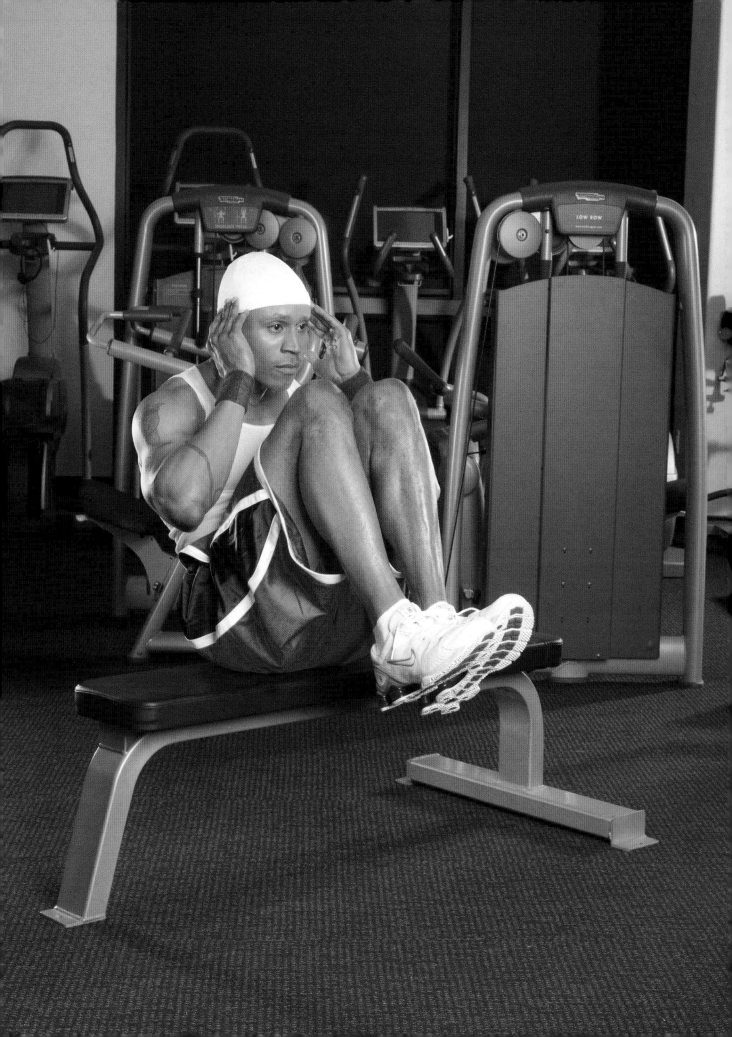

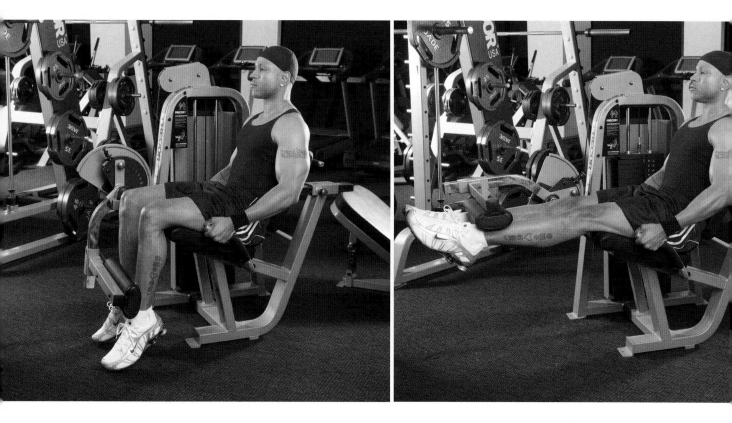

## Leg Extension

1. Set the back pad so your back lies flat against it when your knees are aligned with the machine's axis and the edge of the seat pad tucks snugly behind your knees.

2. Sit down and place your feet under the ankle pad to that it rests where your shins meet your ankles. Grab the side handles. This is the start position.

3. Keep your torso erect and your back against the pad as you extend your legs up toward you, exhaling as you go. Don't thrust so hard that you lose control—slower is better than faster—and don't lock out your knees at the top.

4. In a controlled manner, let the ankle pads back down to the start position, inhaling as you go.

5. Don't let the plates rest on the stack at the bottom. The transition back up should be almost instantaneous.

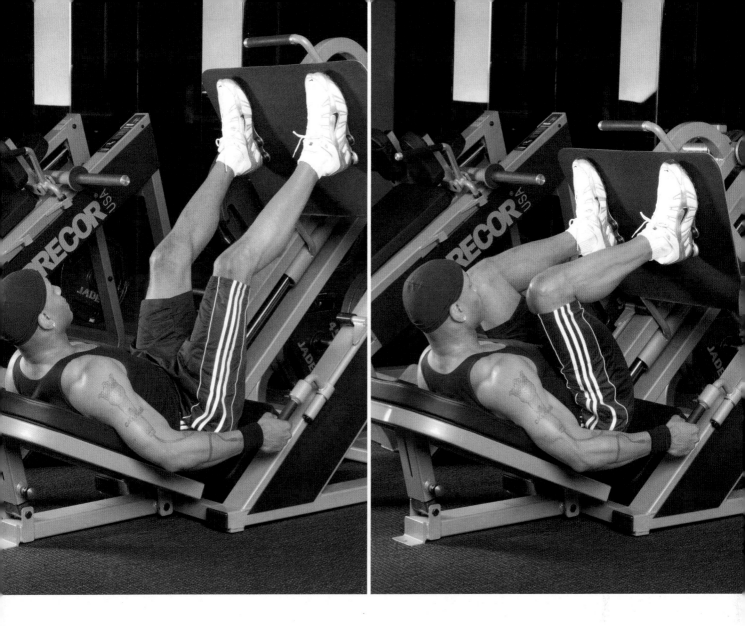

## Leg Press

1. Sit in the machine and adjust the back support to a comfortable position.

2. Place your feet shoulder-width apart on the platform and straighten your legs. Release the locks on the side of the machine to allow the sled to travel up and down unimpeded. This is the start position.

3. Bend your knees to lower the sled, inhaling during the descent.

4. Once your knees approach your shoulders, exhale as you push through the balls of your feet to press the sled back up nearly to full extension. Don't lock out your knees.

5. Keep your back flat against the seat support and your feet flat on the platform throughout.

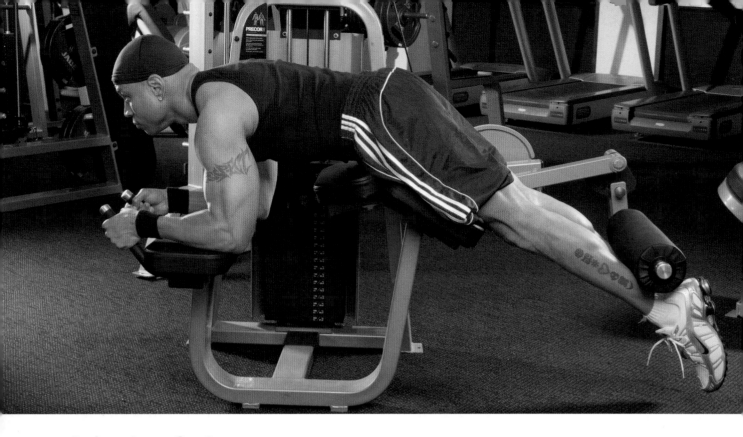

## Lying Leg Curl
1. Lie facedown on the leg-curl machine so that your knees are situated at the end of the seat pad and the rollers rest atop your Achilles tendons.

2. Grasp the handles for support. This is the start position.

3. Smoothly curl your ankles toward your butt, stopping 2 inches from the back of your thighs. (Don't jerk the weight up or allow your hips to rise from the seat pad.) Give your hamstrings an extra squeeze.

4. Exhale on the way up, and then inhale as you lower the ankle pads back to the start position.

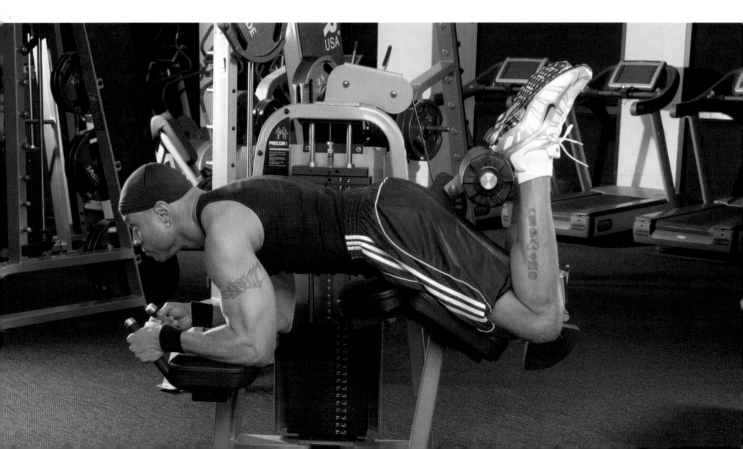

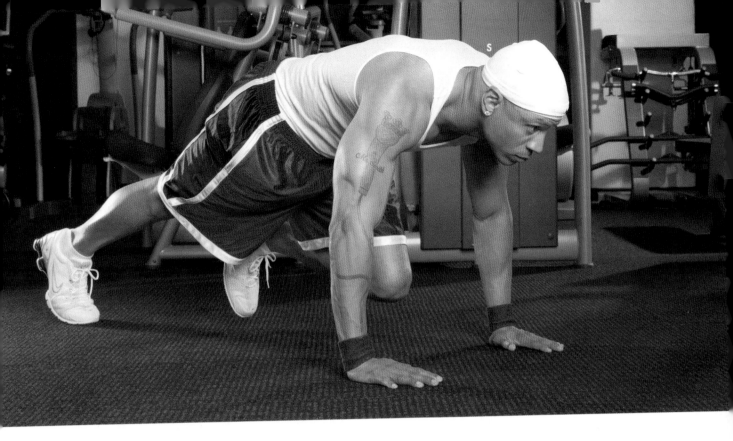

## Mountain Climber
1. Assume a pushup position.

2. In one smooth motion, bring your left knee toward your chest on the same side.

3. Without hesitating, bring your right leg forward while extending your left leg back.

4. Continue in alternating fashion, running on the floor like an Olympic sprinter. Keep your back straight and in line and go for that finish line!

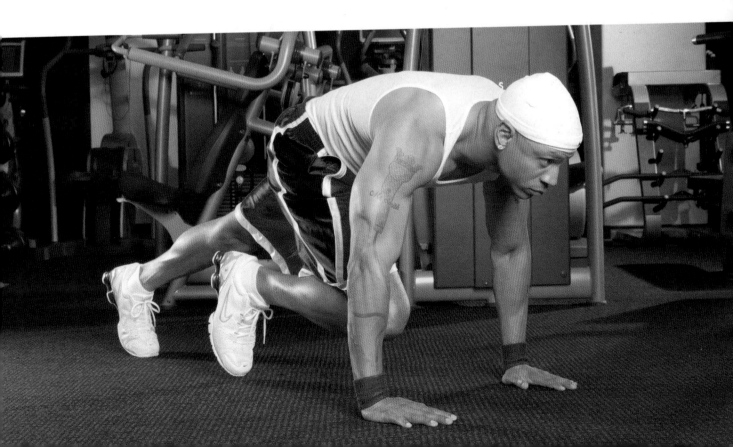

# One-Arm Dumbbell Row

1. Put your left knee and left hand up on a flat bench so that your head looks forward, your back is straight, and your right leg is extended behind you, planted for balance.

2. Grab a dumbbell in your right hand using a thumbless grip. This is the start position.

3. Keeping your torso fixed—don't swing—pull the dumbbell up toward your hip as if you're sawing a piece of wood. Feel a nice squeeze in your back.

4. Return to the start position.

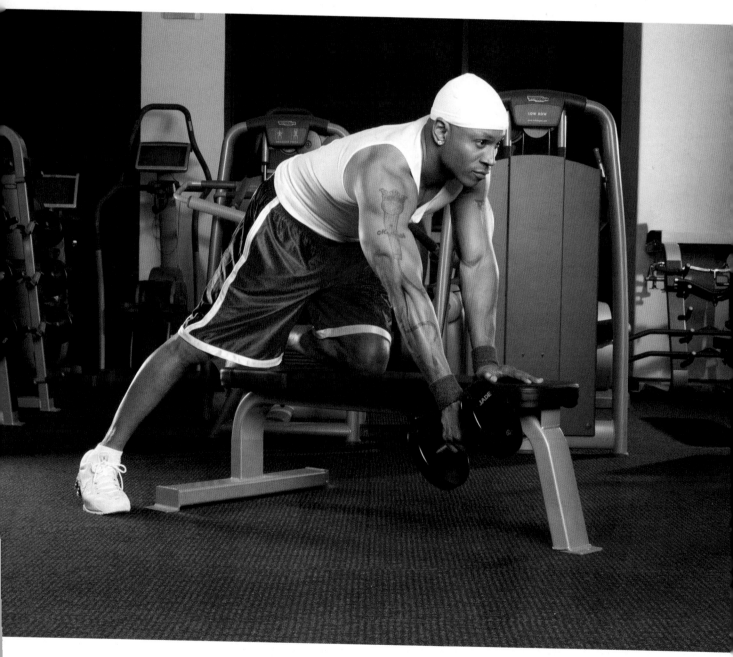

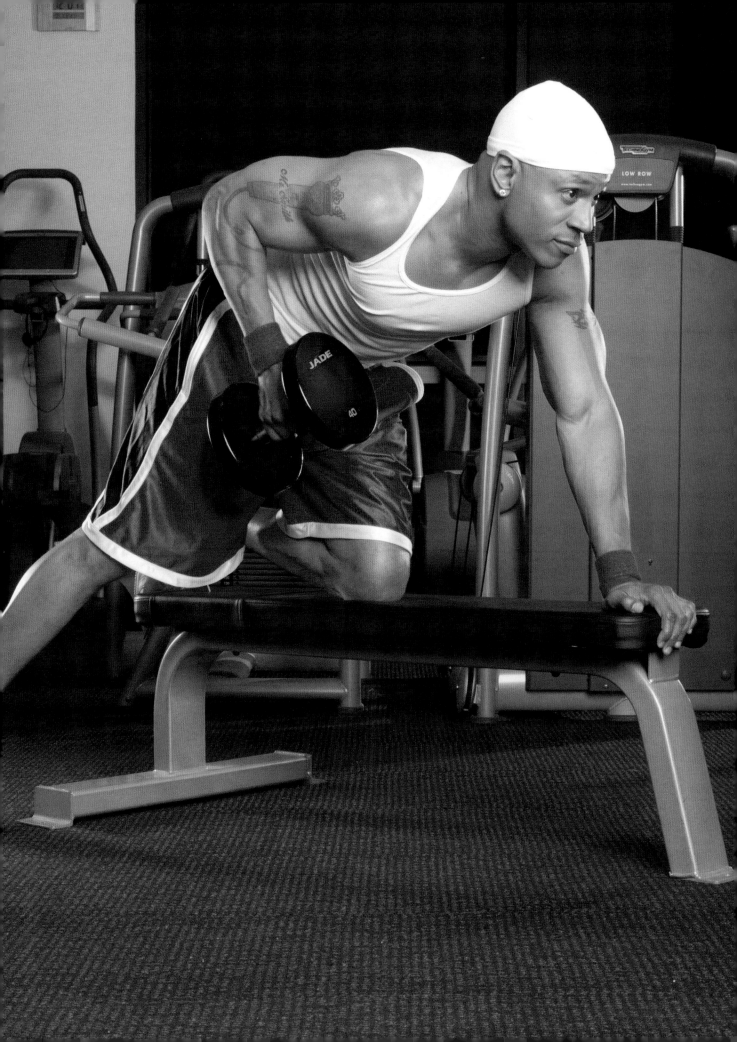

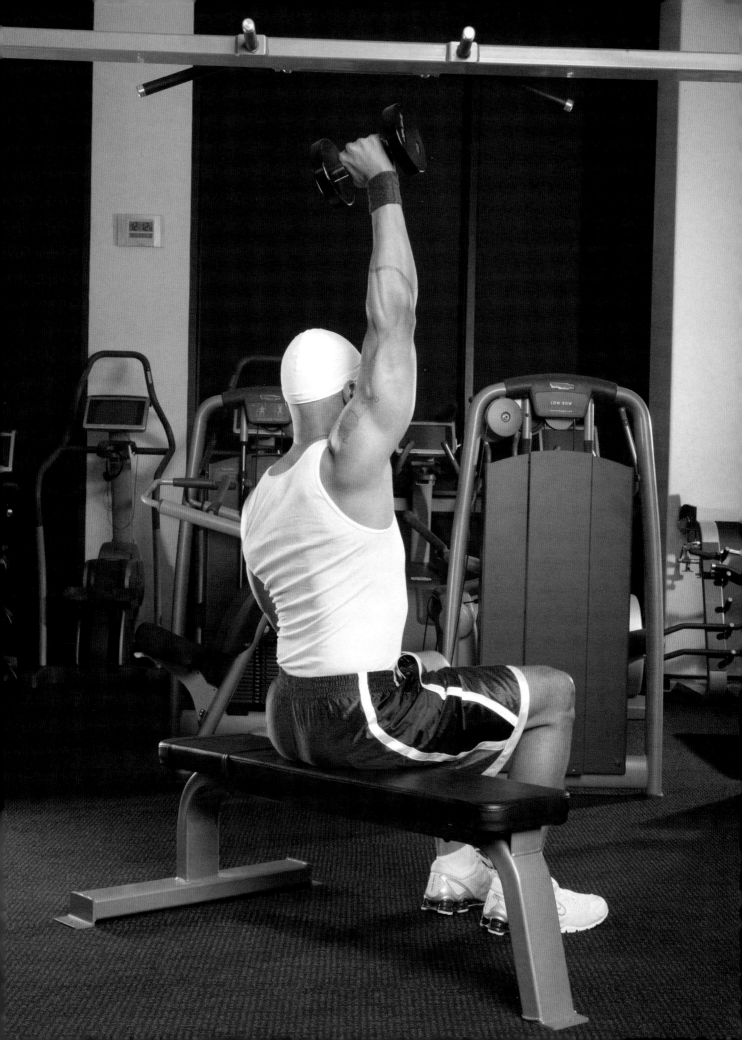

# Overhead Dumbbell Extension

1. Either sit on a bench or stand holding a dumbbell in one hand so that your palm is flush against the inside of one of the plates.

2. Raise the weight overhead to full extension so that your arm passes next to your head and points straight up. This is the start position.

3. Bend your elbow to lower the weight behind your head, getting a full stretch in the triceps at the bottom. Your forearm should be parallel with the floor at this point.

4. Return to the start position, exhaling on the way up.

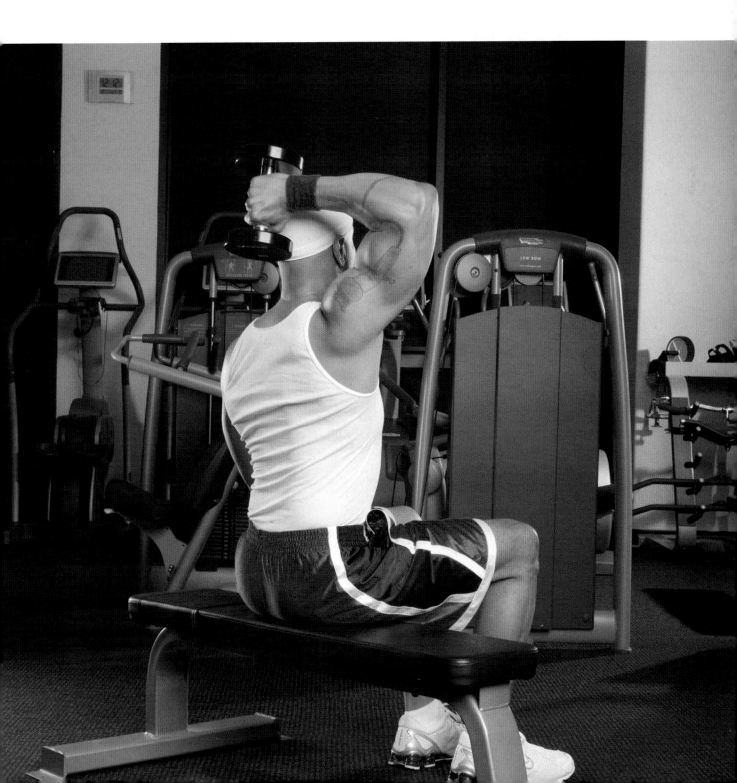

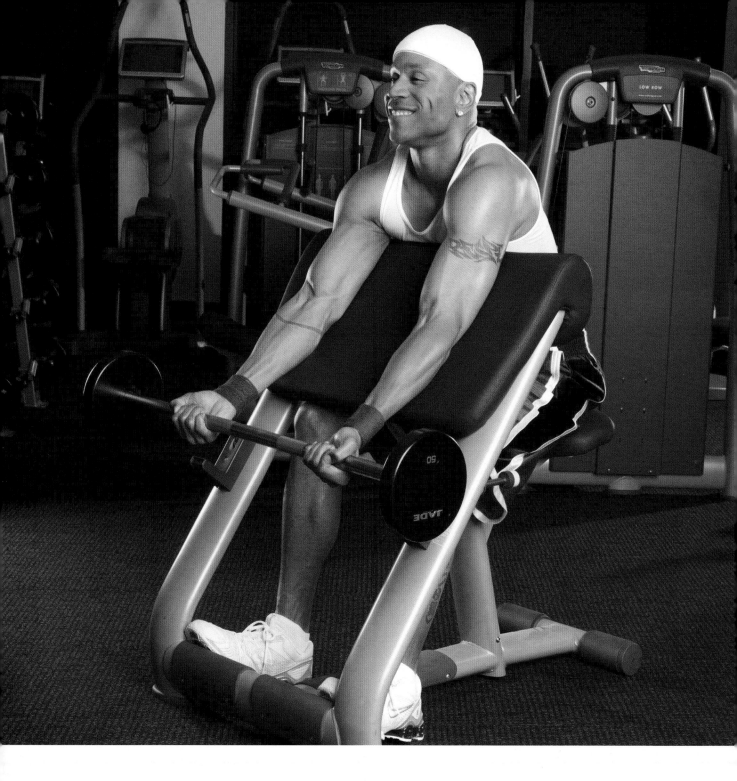

# Preacher Curl

1. Adjust the seat so that the top of the vertically angled pad is at chest height when you're sitting down. Do so—sit down, that is.

2. Plant your feet on the floor or the machine frame, reach down and grasp the bar with an underhand grip, locking your wrists so that they are in line with your forearm. Make sure the top of the pad rests snugly against your underarms. This is the start position.

3. Keeping your body position tight—no momentum—raise the bar up to the front of your shoulders, keeping your triceps in contact with the pad at all times. (As you curl, push your underarms into the pad.) Exhale on the ascent. Squeeze your guns at the top. Pow!

4. Lower the weight to the start position without letting your biceps relax. Inhale on the descent.

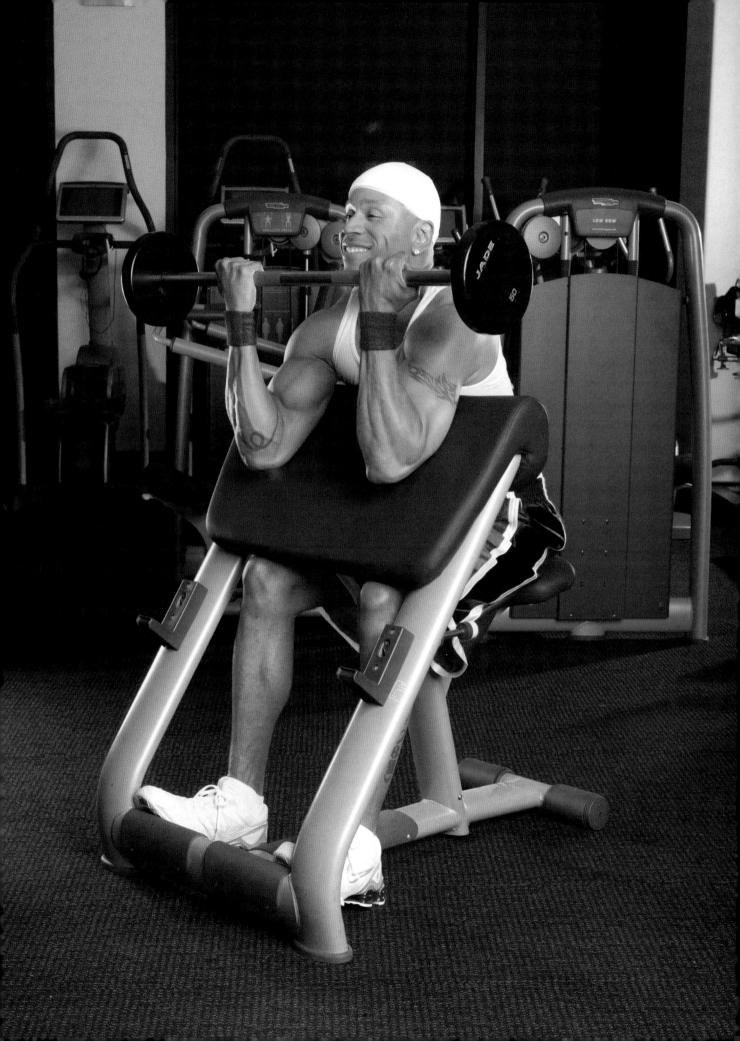

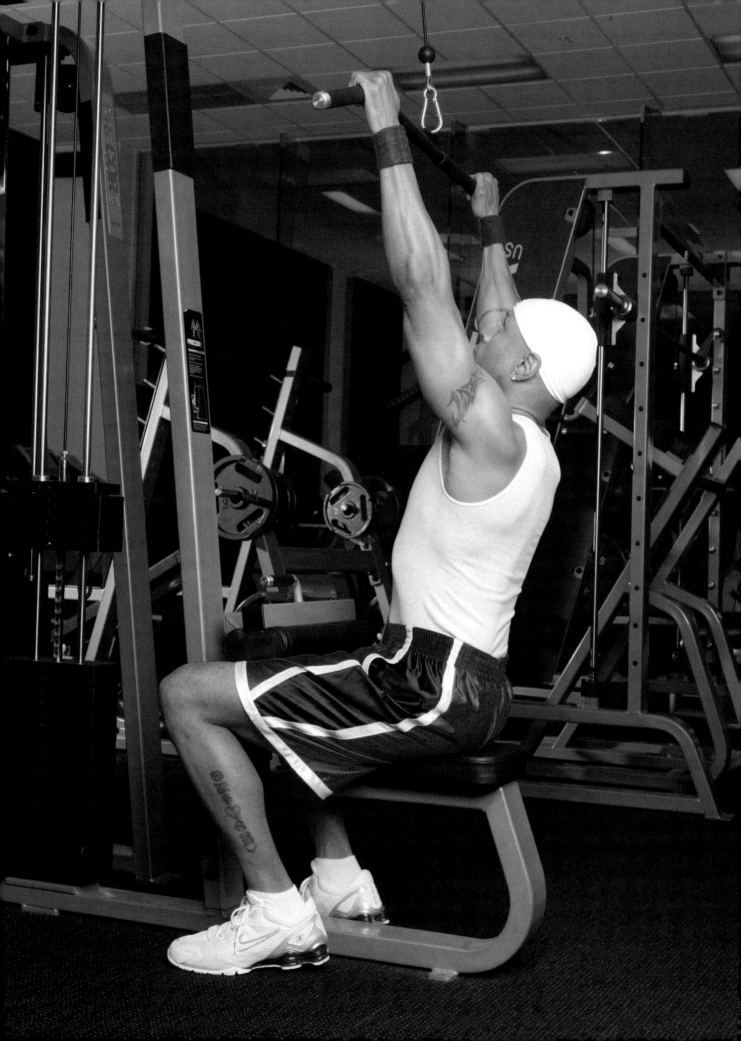

# Pulldown

1. Attach the wide bar to the high pulley.

2. Sit upright on the pad, chest slightly arched, grasping the bar with a thumbless grip so that your arms are almost fully extended. (Hands equal hooks on this exercise.) This is the start position.

3. Keeping your chest arched, exhale as you pull the bar down to your upper chest, thinking about pinching a quarter between your shoulder blades.

4. Pull your elbows back at the bottom and hold for a two-count.

5. Release the muscle contraction and begin inhaling, allowing your arms to return to the start position.

6. Do not let the weight stack swing your body on this exercise. Squeeze every rep like a sponge full of water and eventually NASA will use your back for a launching pad.

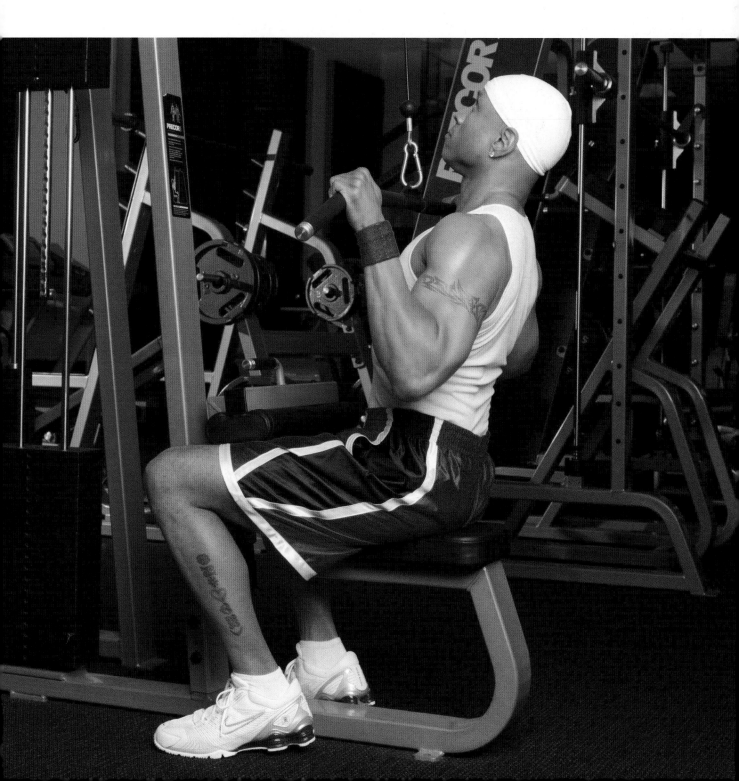

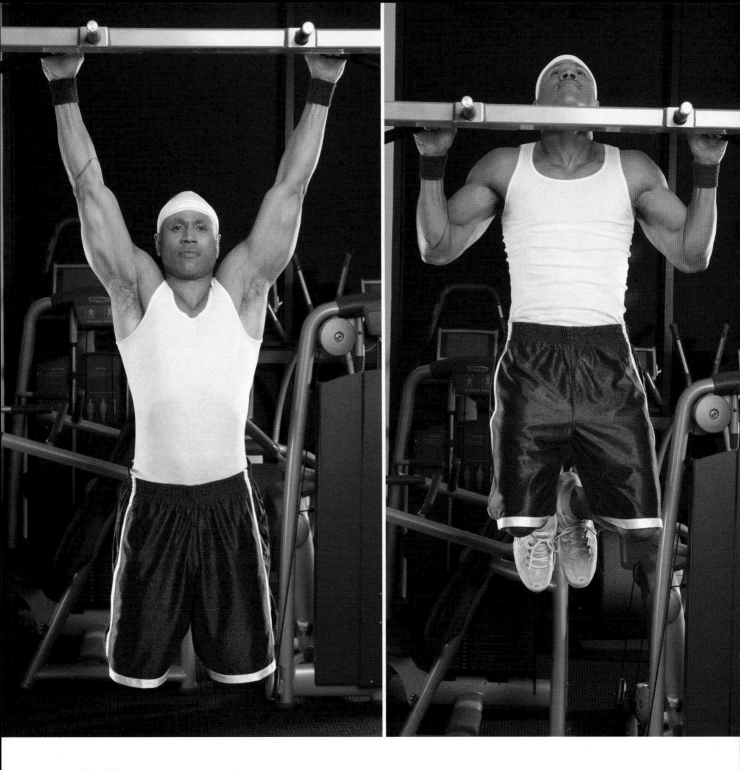

**Pullup** 1. This is one of the most feared exercises in the world. Grasp the bar with an overhand grip, and then hang from it with your body fully extended. This is the start position.

2. Take a deep breath and then exhale as you pull up your body toward the bar, arching your back and bringing your elbows down to your rib cage as you rise. Stop crying and just do it!

3. Lower your body back to the start position.

4. This is a hard exercise, and if you can't complete the assigned number of reps, use the assisted pullup machine if your gym has one. The way those work is that you set the pin to select a weight that will offset some of your body weight. Now go to work!

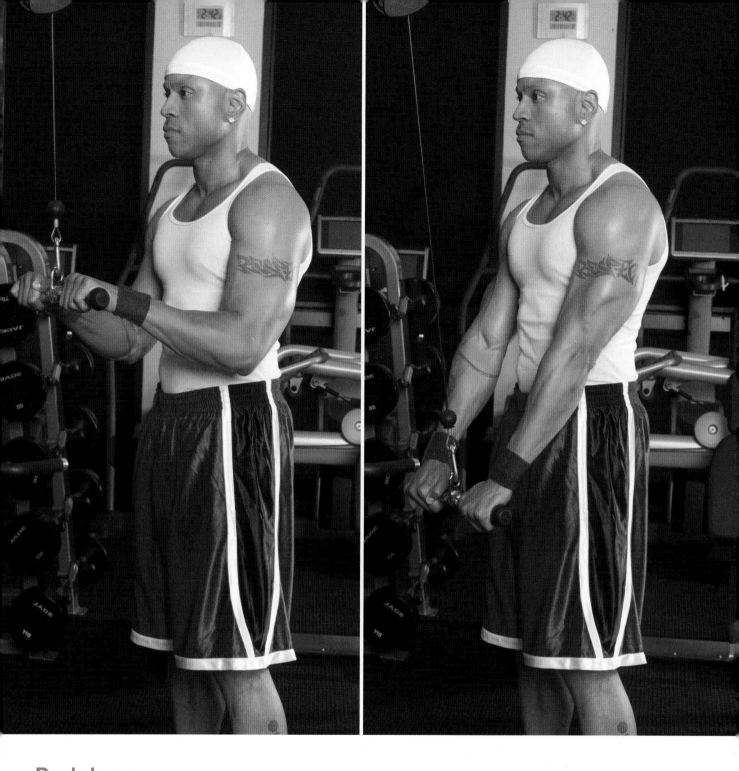

# Pushdown

1. Attach a straight or angled bar to a high pulley.

2. Stand facing the stack and grasp the bar overhand so your thumbs sit 8 to 10 inches apart. Stand tall with your feet planted shoulder-width apart. This is the start position.

3. Press down the bar until your arms are fully extended, keeping your elbows tucked into your sides, chest up, shoulders back, abs tight.

4. Inhale on the way up and exhale on the way down. Don't lean over the bar, and don't use momentum.

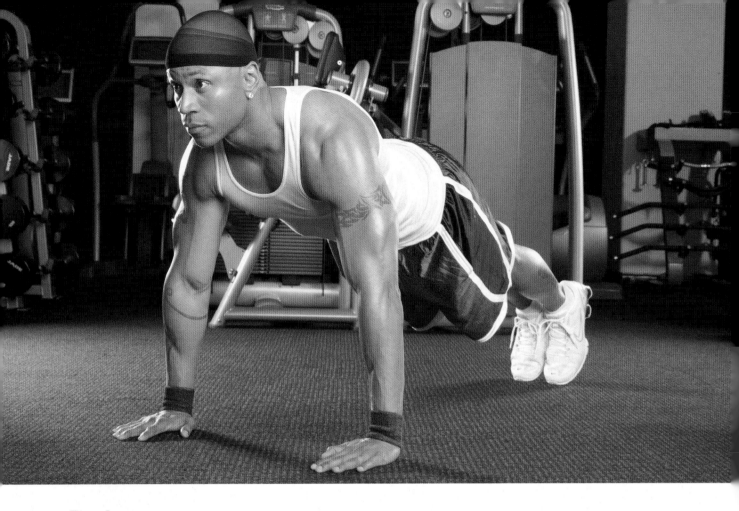

## Pushup

1. Time to return to gym class—only this time you're coached by a rap star and his trainer, not a gym coach with elastic shorts two sizes too small, a whistle dangling around his neck, and a dinged-up powder-blue van filled with soccer balls and orange cones out in the parking lot.

2. Assume a classic pushup position: back flat, body straight, hands spaced slightly wider than your shoulders and underneath them, eyes looking straight ahead, arms fully extended, balance provided by your palms and toes.

3. Bend your elbows to lower your torso until your chest is just 1 inch from the floor. Inhale. Feel a deep stretch at the bottom. Don't let your butt sag below your body.

4. Push back up to return to the start position. Exhale during the ascent.

5. To make the move more difficult, scissor-kick one of your legs up as you rise to full arm extension, as shown at right.

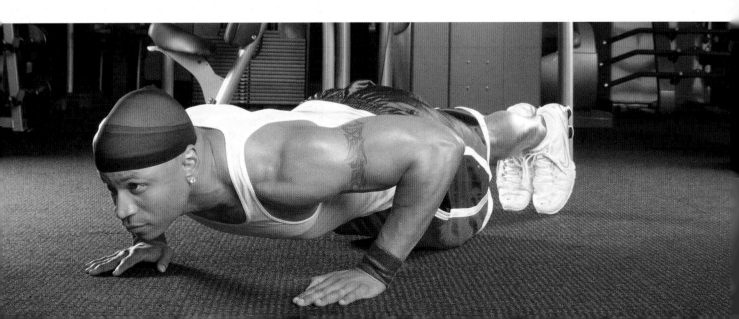

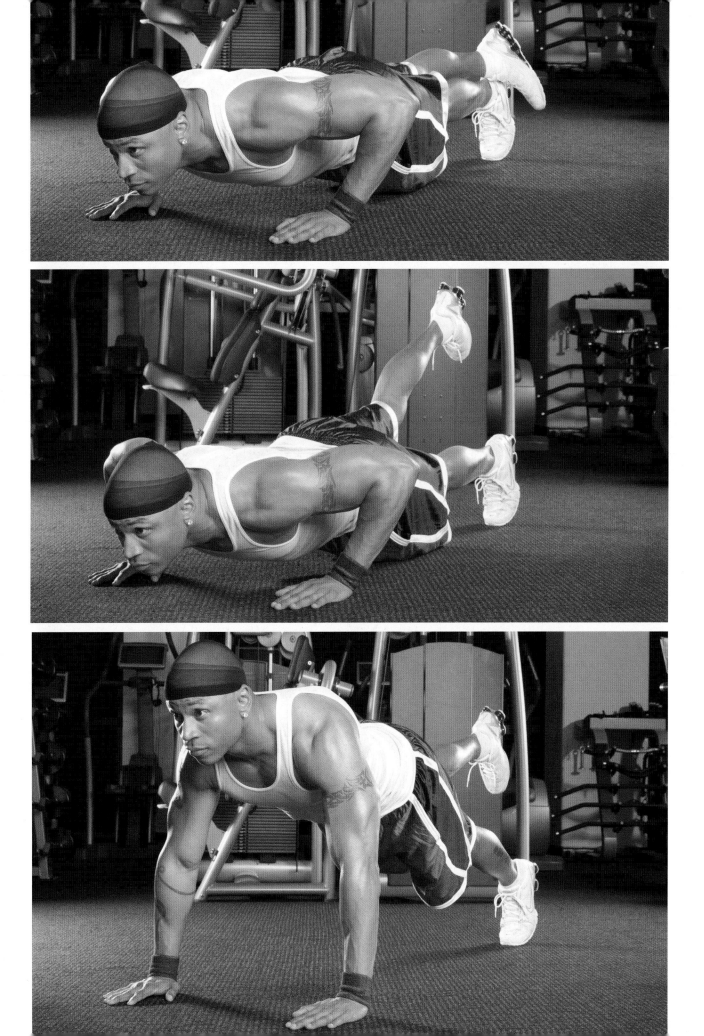

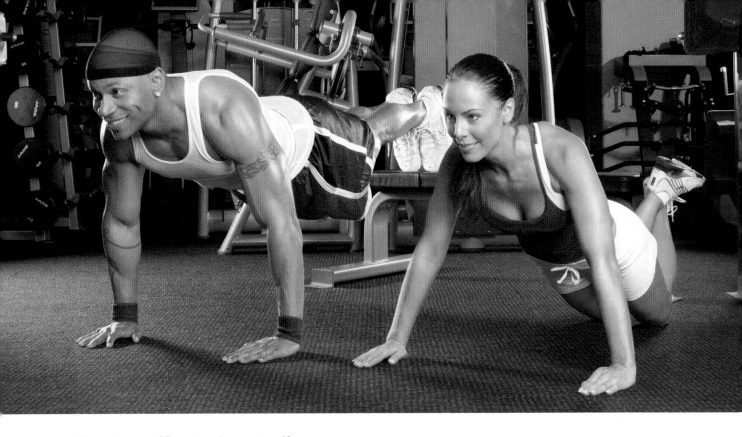

## Pushup (feet elevated)

1. Assume a pushup position—back flat, body straight, hands shoulder-width apart, eyes looking ahead, arms fully extended—but place your feet on a bench 12 to 16 inches off the floor.

2. Bend your elbows to lower your torso until your chest is 1 inch from the floor. Feel a deep stretch at the bottom. Inhale during the descent.

3. Push back up to return to the start position. Exhale during the ascent.

4. If this pushup is too difficult, start with your knees on the floor and progress from there.

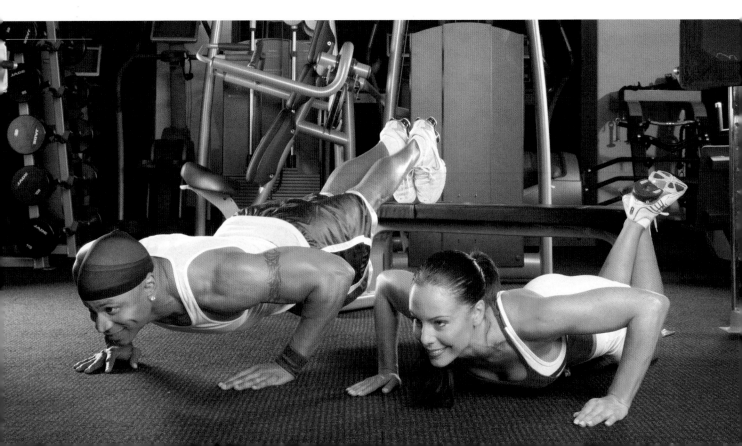

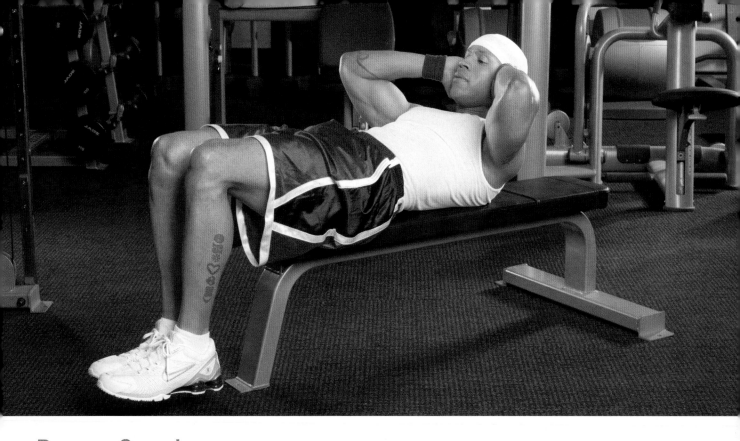

## Reverse Crunch

1. Lie flat on a bench or the floor and raise your thighs till they point straight up while keeping your shins horizontal, so your knees are bent 90 degrees. This is the start position.

2. Simultaneously draw in your abs as you roll your pelvis toward your torso, stopping only after your hips leave the bench or floor and your knees come over your chest. Exhale during the roll.

3. Return to the start position, inhaling.

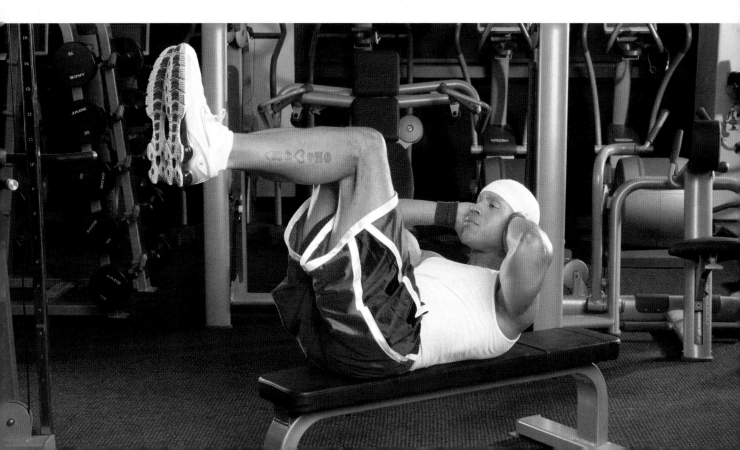

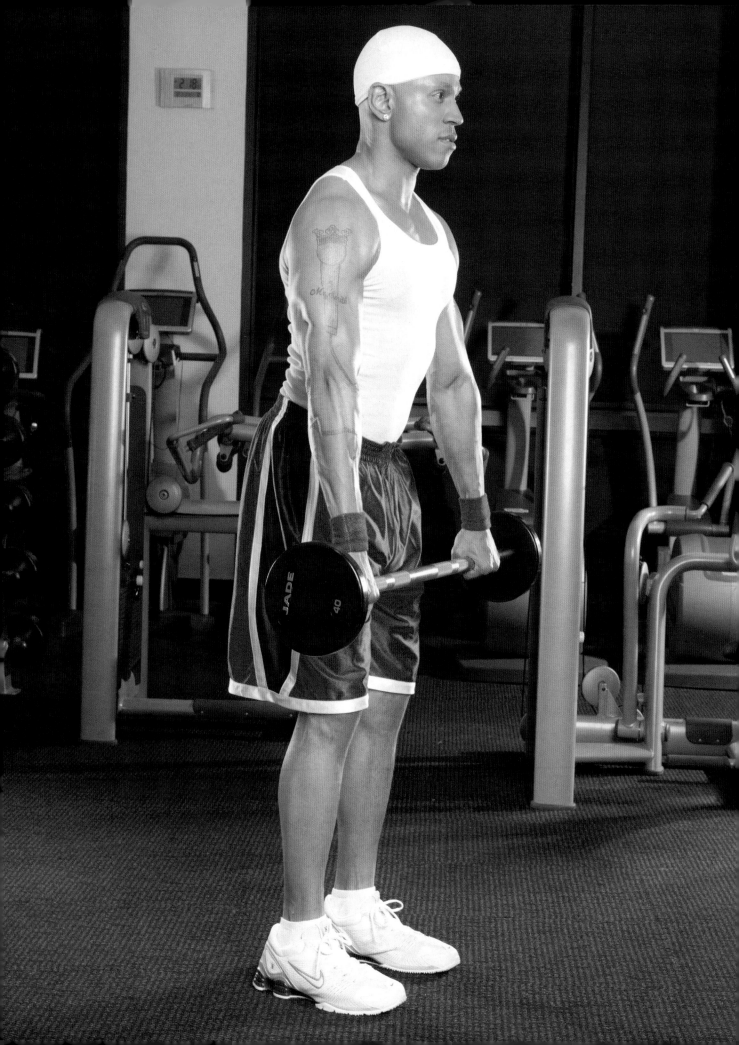

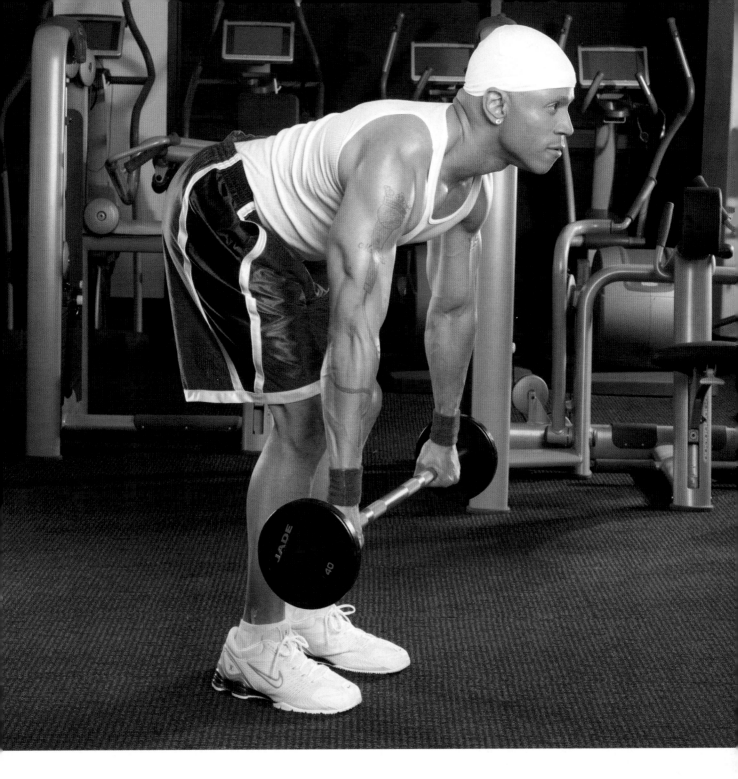

# Romanian Deadlift

1. Remove a weighted barbell from a squat rack or bench and stand holding it overhand at arms' length, hands and feet shoulder-width apart. (Start with a light weight until you've perfected the technique. Then go heavier.)

2. Bend your knees slightly. This is the start position.

3. Keeping your back flat (no rounding!) and your gaze fixed forward, bend at the waist and drop your butt back to lower the bar in a slow and deliberate movement until your torso is about parallel with the floor.

4. Push through your heels to return to the start position. Don't lock out your back at the top.

5. Inhale as you descend and exhale coming back up.

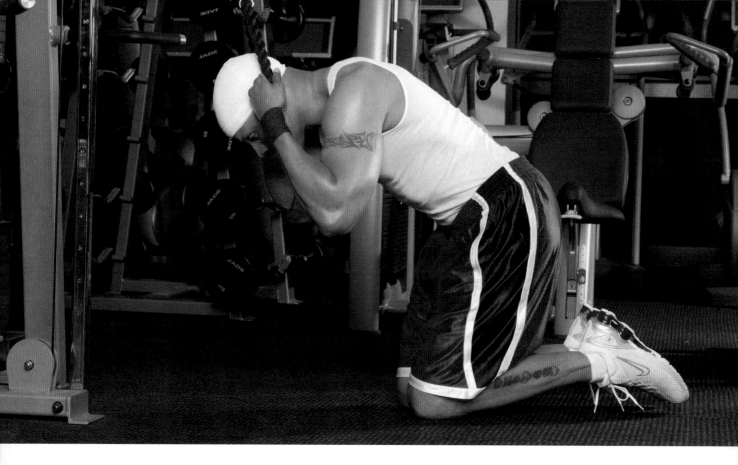

## Rope Crunch

1. Hang a bifurcated rope attachment from the high pulley of a cable stack.

2. Grasp the rope handle with both hands, which should be next to your ears. Tuck your chin. This is the start position.

3. Without letting your hands slip away from the side of your head, curl your shoulders forward in a semicircle toward your knees until your elbows almost touch them. Contract your abs and exhale.

4. Return to the start position.

5. The pace throughout should be slow and deliberate, not fast.

6. Don't lower your hips—you'll know you have when your butt touches your heels.

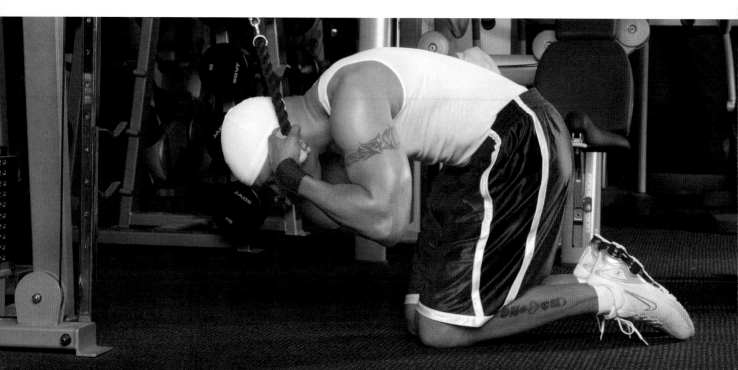

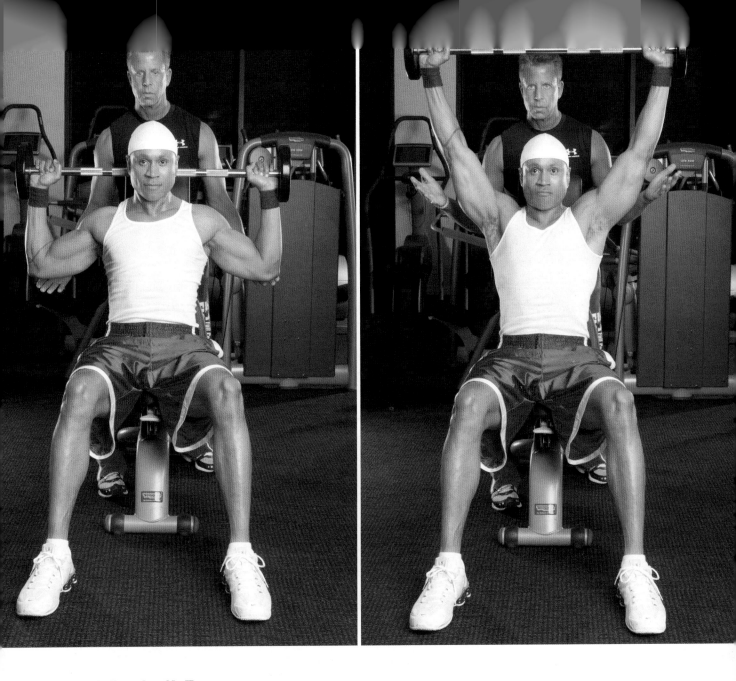

## Seated Barbell Press

1. Sit on a bench with a back support perpendicular with the seat pad. (If your gym doesn't have such a bench, be extra vigilant when it comes to keeping your back straight.)

2. Space your feet evenly on the floor. Pick up a barbell and raise it to shoulder height so that it rests behind your head, palms facing forward. This is the start position.

3. Press the barbell overhead until your arms are fully extended. Exhale as you press, and don't lean forward, or you risk straining your neck.

4. Return to the start position, inhaling on the way down.

## Seated Cable Row

1. Walk over to the seated cable machine, with all the little square weight plates stacked up. Well, what are you waiting for—sit down!

2. Assume an upright position with your back slightly arched, holding the small handles in front of you at arms' length. (If some big dude is using them, walk over to him and explain that you're doing the Platinum Workout and that you need those handles. He will quickly give them to you.) This is the start position.

3. Take a deep breath and then exhale as you pull the handles to a point 2 inches below the pit of your stomach, drawing together your shoulder blades.

4. Here's where it gets tricky: Let the handle travel back to the start position under control, never losing the arch in your back, even at full extension. You're in charge; don't let them pull you. (We don't want you flying headfirst into the weight stack.) Extend your arms fully, only don't roll your shoulders forward; keep them back.

5. Remember the guy who looked like he could move mountains, the one who gave you the handles? He finished the Platinum Workout 3 weeks ago.

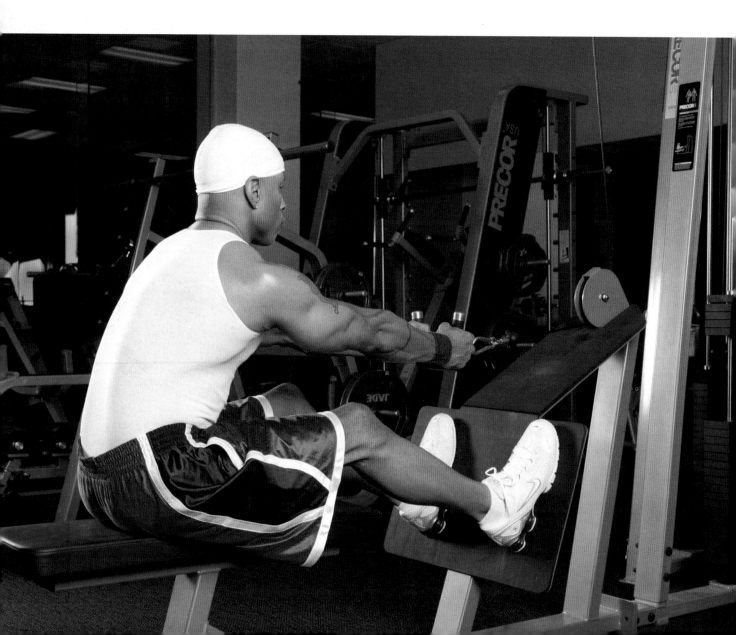

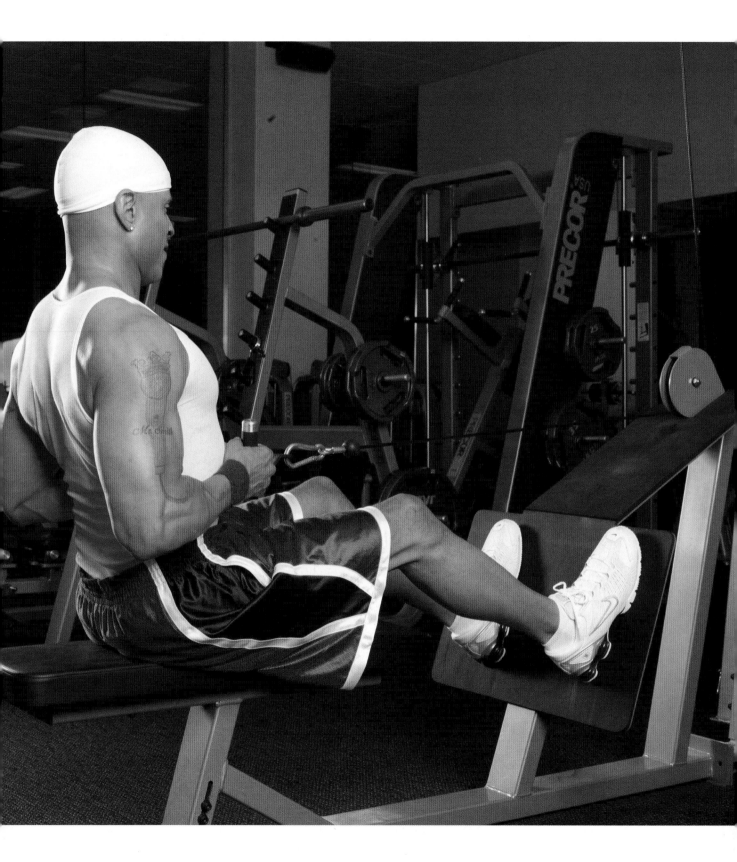

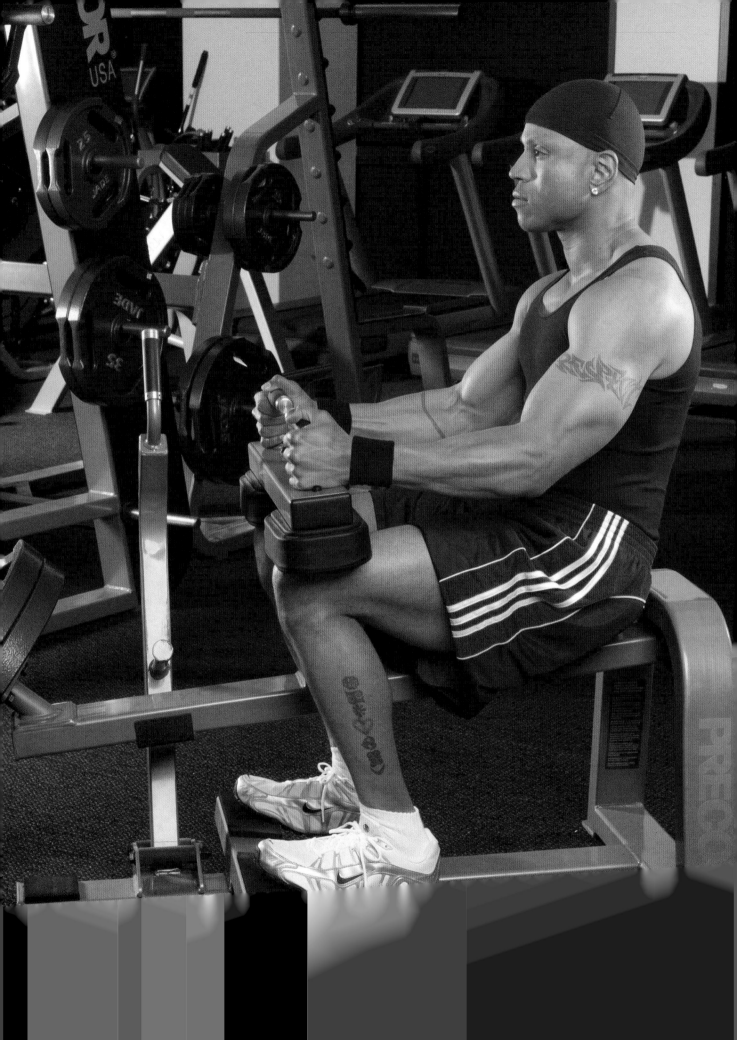

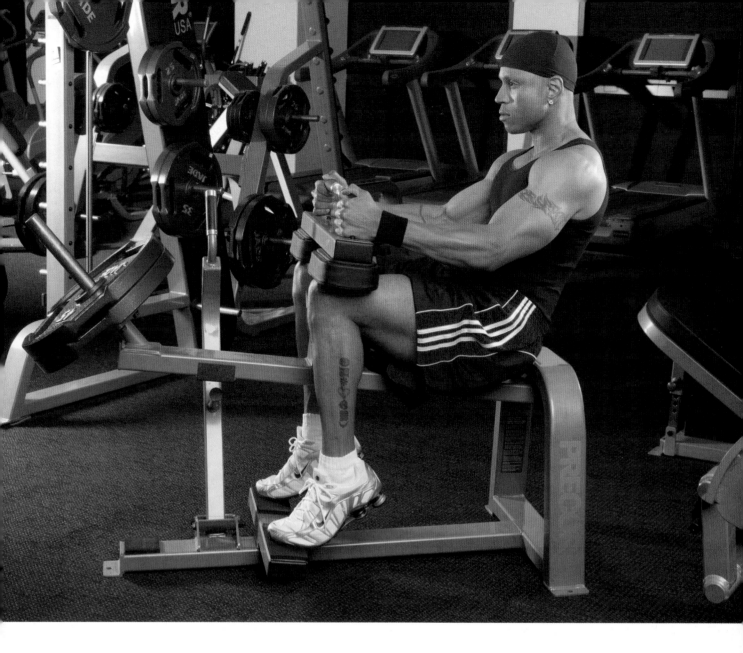

## Seated Calf Raise
1. Sit on the machine and adjust the thigh pad so it fits snugly on your lower thighs, just above the knees.

2. Place your feet 12 inches apart and rest on the balls, not the heels. Lift the handle to release the weight. This is the start position.

3. Deliberately and under control, lower your heels, which are free-floating, until your calves feel fully stretched. Inhale on the descent.

4. Push up on the balls of your foot to a fully extended position. Don't bounce; let your calves do the work. Exhale on the ascent and you're good to go.

# SCOOTER'S *FAT-BURNING TIP*

If you can't get to the gym when traveling, use the hotel stairwell. Walk up two flights, do pushups on the landing, walk up two more flights, jump rope, walk up two more flights hitting every other step, and then do body-weight squats. Go back to your room and get a massage.

## Seated Dumbbell Press (not pictured)

1. Sit on a bench with a back support perpendicular with the seat pad. (If your gym doesn't have such a bench, be extra vigilant when it comes to keeping your back straight.)

2. Space your feet evenly on the floor. Pick up the dumbbells positioned on either side of you and raise them to shoulder height, palms facing forward. Press your back firmly against the back pad. This is the start position.

3. Press the dumbbells overhead, bringing them close together at the top without actually letting them touch. Exhale as you press, and don't lean forward, or you risk straining your neck.

4. Arc your elbows down to return to the start position, inhaling on the way down. Now work!

I look back on Venus
I look back on Mars
And **I burn with the fire**
**Of ten million stars**

—LL Cool J, **"10 Million Stars," 2003**

**Skull-Crusher (not pictured)** 1. Don't think for 1 minute that the name tells you what to do, or you'll be in serious trouble. Don't worry—we gotcha covered.

2. Sit down on a flat bench holding a weighted EZ-curl bar across your thighs using an overhand grip, so that 6 to 8 inches separate your thumbs.

3. Raise it to arms' length overhead as you lie down, so that you're staring straight up at it. Plant your feet on the floor. This is the start position.

4. Keeping your upper arms set near the sides of your head throughout this exercise, bend your elbows to lower the bar slowly down to your hairline (or at least what used to be your hairline) or slightly behind your head—whichever groove feels better to you. As we begin our descent, inhale—no gas mask required.

5. At the bottom, your elbows should be ready to kiss the sky, as Jimi would say.

6. Extend your arms in a semicircular motion to return the bar to the start position. Exhale on the way up. Keep your wrists locked tight and locked, and your upper arms parallel with each other.

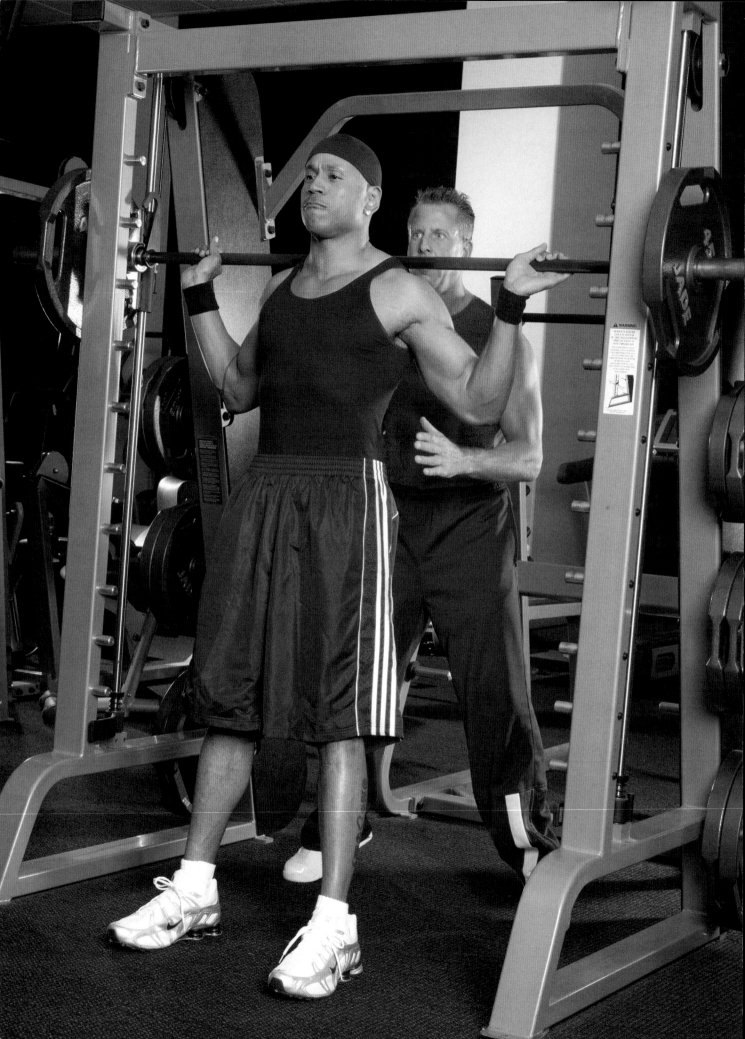

# Smith Machine Squat

1. Step under the bar in a Smith machine squat rack with your feet parallel to each other, shoulder-width apart. Grasp the bar with an overhand grip so it rests across your traps.

2. Unhook the safety latches and straighten up with your chest high, shoulder blades squeezed back, gaze fixed forward. This is the start position.

3. Bend your knees as if sitting down in a chair, making sure that your knees stay aligned with your feet, until your thighs reach parallel with the floor.

4. Push up through your feet without bouncing to return to the start position. Avoid locking out your knees at the top. Remember to rehook the bar at set's end.

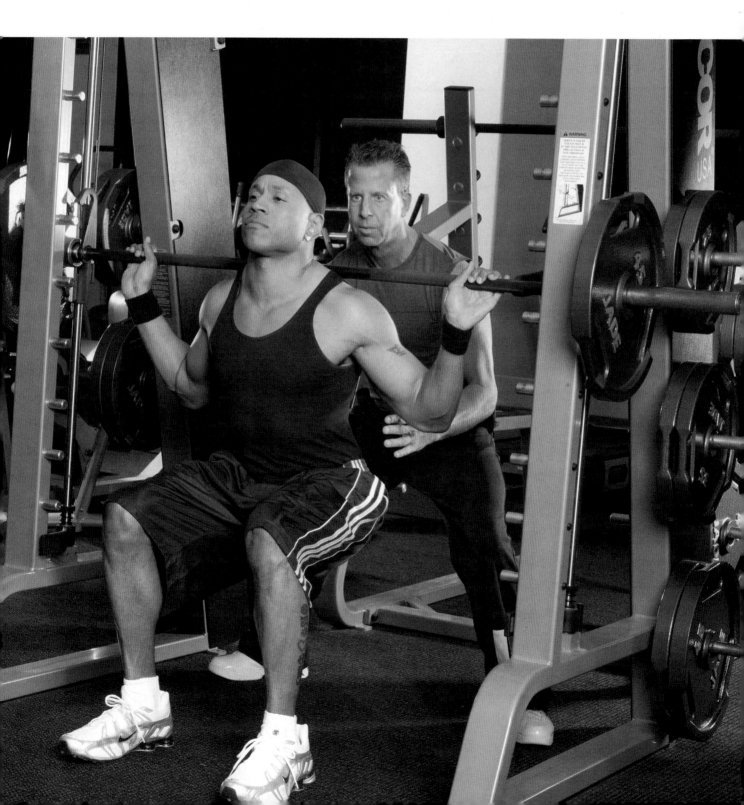

## Squat (body weight only)

1. Stand with your chest high, shoulder blades squeezed back, gaze fixed forward and a smile on your face, arms extended in front of you, feet parallel to each other, shoulder-width apart. This is the start position.

2. Bend your knees as if sitting down in a chair, making sure that your knees stay aligned with your feet, until your thighs reach parallel with the floor.

3. Push up through your feet without bouncing to return to the start position.

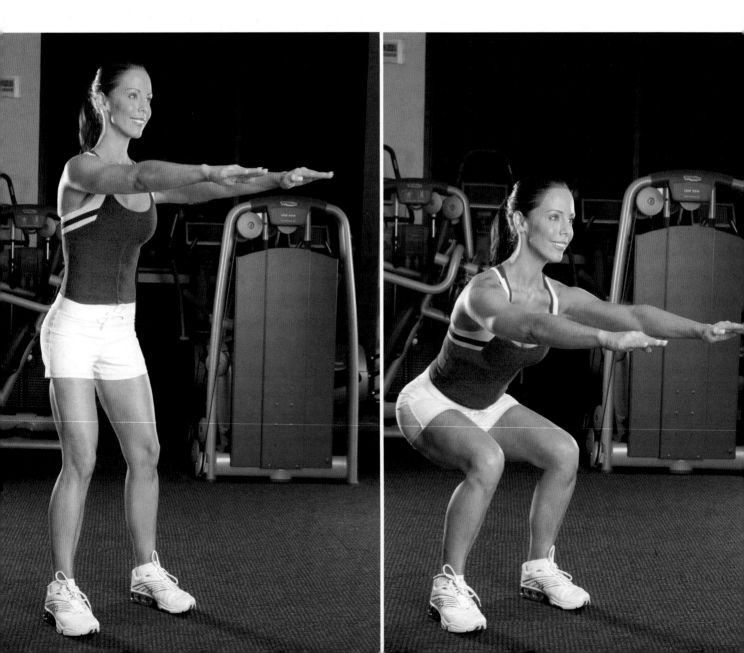

# Sprinting with Tubing

1. Attach rubber tubing to a fixed point, such as a piece of exercise equipment, and then wrap it around your waist. This is the start position.

2. Run as if you're on a track, except the tubing will prevent you from moving forward. It's like running in place, but with resistance applied.

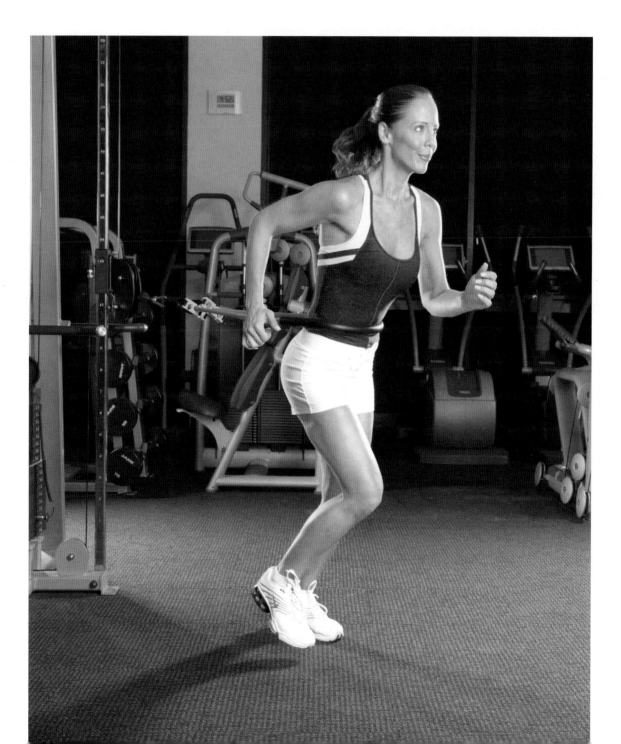

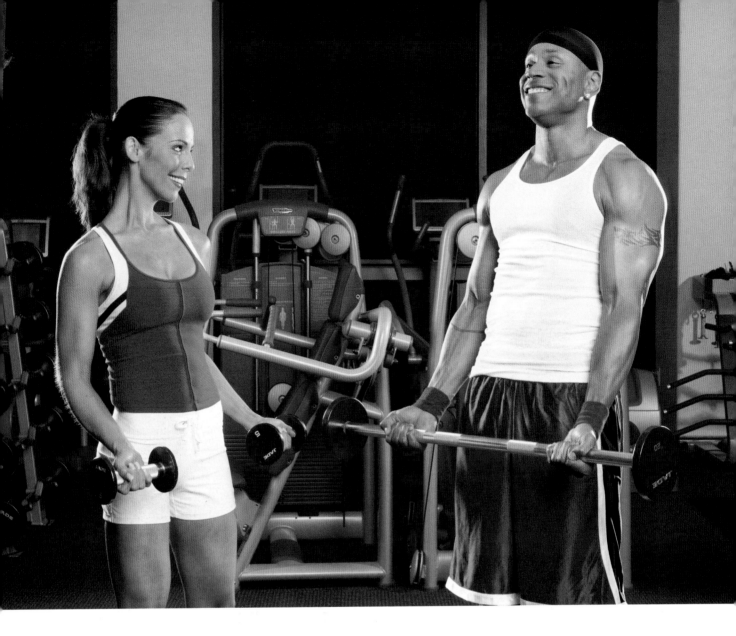

**Standing Barbell Curl** 1. Stand holding a barbell with an underhand grip, hands shoulder-width apart, at arms' length, down by your thighs.

2. Exhale as you curl the bar up to the front of your shoulders.

3. Inhale as you lower it back down.

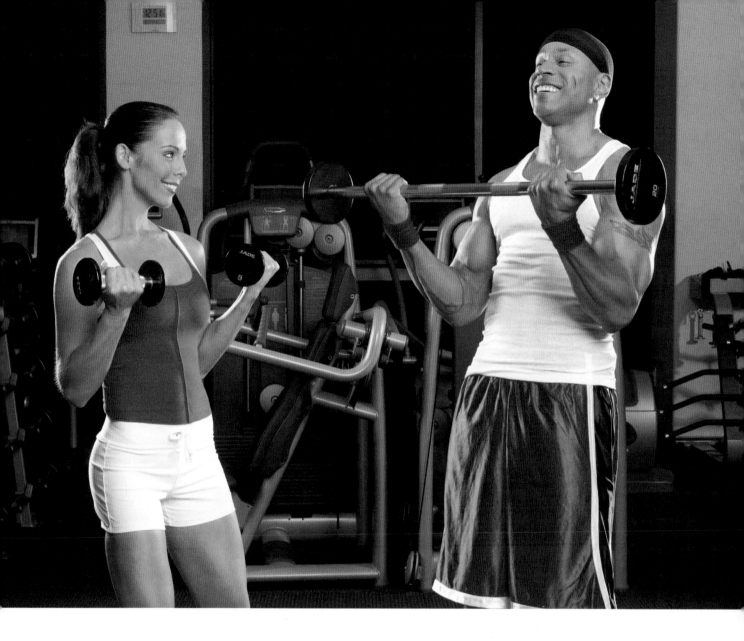

4. Throughout the entire rep, keep your upper arms stationary, more or less pinned against your sides, so that your elbows function like hinges.

5. Don't throw the weight up; move it in a controlled rhythm.

6. Curls can also be done with dumbbells, for variety's sake.

Don't call it a comeback
I been here for years
Rockin' my peers and puttin' suckas in fear
Makin' the tears rain down **like a monsoon**
Listen to the bass go boom
Explosion overpowerin'
Over the competition **i'm towerin'**

—LL Cool J, **"Mama Said Knock You Out," 1990**

**Standing Calf Raise (not pictured)** 1. Stand in or on the machine so the pads rest atop your shoulders, with your feet shoulder-width apart, and the balls of your feet balanced on the edge of the footrests.

2. Stand up straight and release the releases (if the machine has them). This is the start position.

3. In a controlled and deliberate manner, lower your heels, which are free-floating, until your calves feel fully stretched. Inhale on the descent.

4. Push up on the balls of your feet to a fully extended position. Don't bounce or jerk the weight up from your traps; let your calves do the work. Exhale on the ascent.

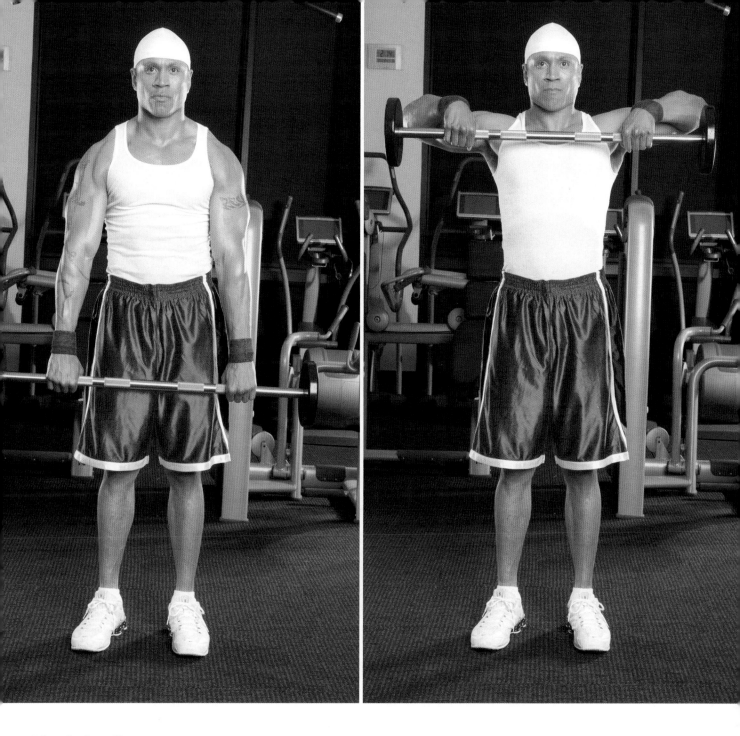

**Upright Row** 1. Stand up straight holding a barbell in front of you at arms' length, using an overhand grip at least shoulder-width apart. This is the start position.

2. Keep the bar close to your body as you exhale and pull it up, flaring your elbows during the ascent.

3. Lower the bar back to the start position. Inhale on the way down.

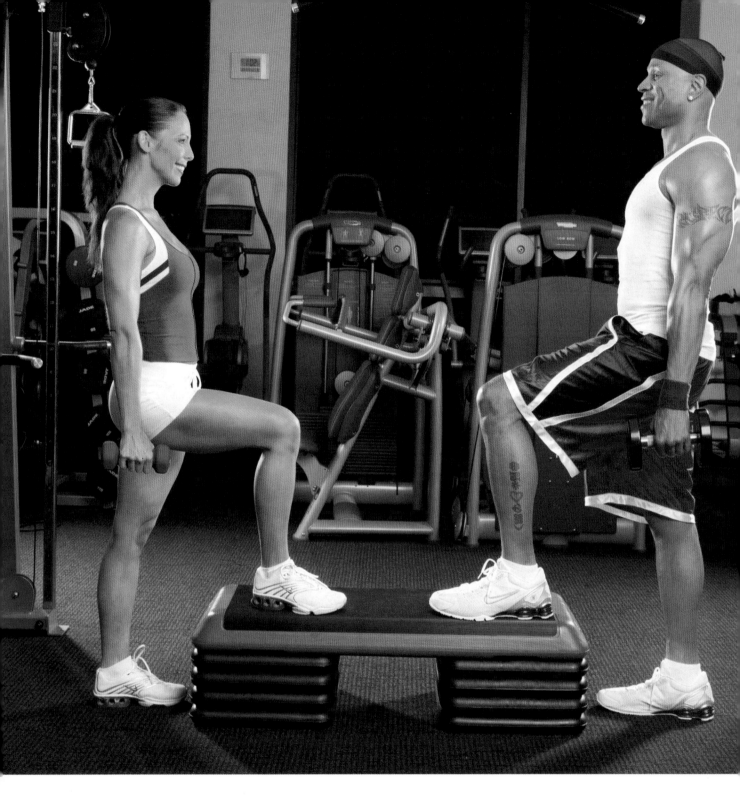

## Stepup

1. Stand upright holding dumbbells at arms' length in front of a box or stacked aerobics steps 15 to 18 inches high. Place one foot up on the bench. The knee of your trailing leg should be slightly bent. This is the start position.

2. Pushing off the leg already on the box, step up onto it with the other leg. Exhale as you step.

3. Step down, removing the lead leg first.

4. Begin your next rep with the opposite foot on the box.

5. Continue in alternating fashion until you've completed all your reps.

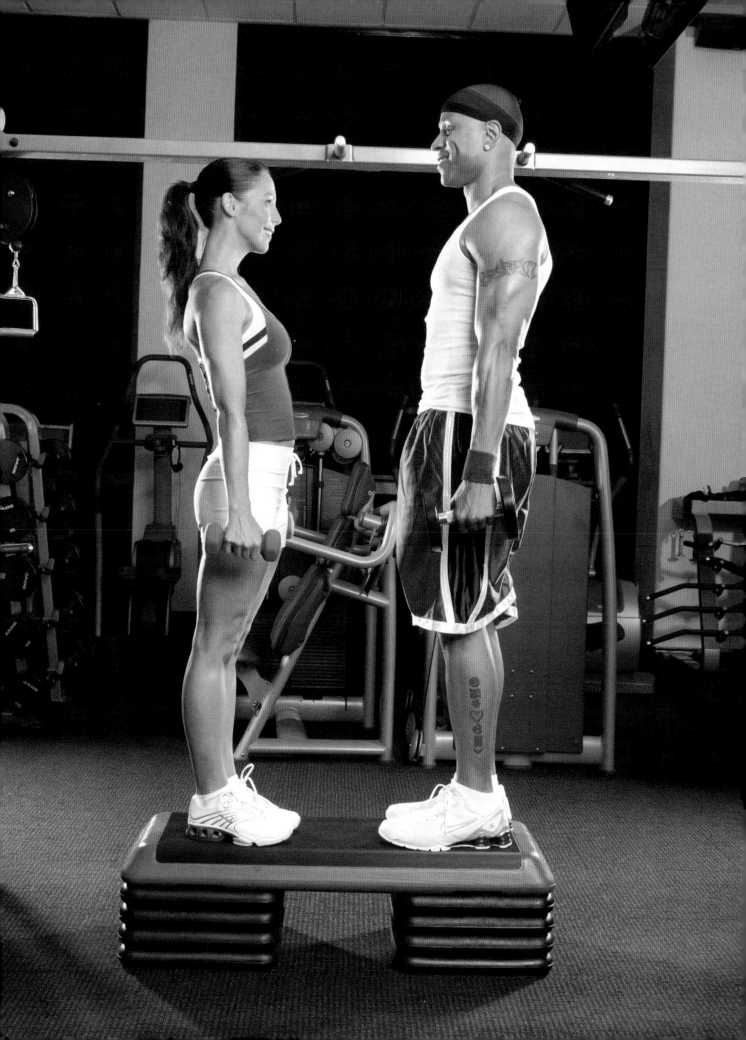

# REEL MUSCLE

**A time line of LL Cool J's career as an actor**

## 1970s

**ON HIS BIGGEST EARLY ACTING INFLUENCE:**
Bruce Lee was a man of few words, but he was in shape, he was strong, he was different, he didn't fit in. I loved him. He was a great inspiration for me. He was a very positive and successful guy on a lot of levels. Think about it from a discipline point of view. This was an Asian actor at a time when no one would think about accepting that, who was so disciplined physically and mentally that he was able to take his life to another level and basically conquer the world. A pretty inspiring guy.

## 1985

**ON HIS MEMORIES OF *KRUSH GROOVE*:**
Being an extra on the set. At that time, I had moved out, I was living at my friend Cornell's house, in the basement, and he would call me up every day from work and say, "Go down to the set!" I'm like, "For what? I don't have a part." He's like, "I don't care—just go down there!" So I'd go down and be an extra, or I'd sweep on set, and I'd just be hangin' and hangin' and hangin', and eventually I got a part. And what had happened, incredibly, was that I overslept when I was supposed to shoot a video for "I Can't Live Without My Radio." As a result, I never shot that video. So the movie became my video. That was the first time the world saw me.

## 1995

**ON *IN THE HOUSE*:**
I used to be around Quincy Jones all the time because I was dating his daughter, and me and him used to kick it a lot and talk about different ideas. That was just an idea that came up, and he wanted to do it, and he did it. That was the first time I learned to wake up every morning and be somewhere on time. At first it was very tough for me. But I'm very proud of *In the House* because I was able to maintain my integrity. We always put out positive messages and positive energy; always used that vehicle to do and say something good. I've grown as an actor since then, obviously, but other than that, when it plays now, it's still putting a positive vibe out there. That's what it's all about.

## 1998

**ON *HALLOWEEN H$_2$O: 20 YEARS LATER*:**
That was the first movie that I did during the second phase of my film career. I had stayed away from film for many years and just focused on music. Then I came back after the TV show, and this was the first movie I did.

## 1999

**ON *DEEP BLUE SEA*:**
The most appealing role I've ever had. It was fun, it was crazy, it was a success from the beginning, and my role just kept getting bigger and bigger on that set. They actually had to reshoot the ending so I could survive because the people [in test screenings] didn't want me to die.

**ON** *ANY GIVEN SUNDAY*:

It was a dream-fulfilling experience because growing up I had always wanted to be a pro football player. And if I had stayed on Long Island, I probably would have pursued it more vigorously. I actually got to run with the ball in Texas Stadium, wearing No. 33—and [Tony] Dorsett was the guy that I loved growing up—and I got to play on a team and run the ball and take some real hits. It was great.

## 2002

**ON** *ROLLERBALL*:

This is the movie that encouraged me to get in shape, period. I looked at the screen and said to myself, *You can do better.* I wasn't myself. I was put in a second position, and I didn't feel like I looked like I should be in the first position. You can't be No. 2, looking like you're supposed to be No. 2, mad you're not No. 1. You shouldn't be No. 2, upset that you're No. 2, when you look, act, and operate like you should be No. 2, and the only thing that wants to be No. 1 is your ego. Plus, I felt like it was a bad movie. Wack. Terrible. That's the thing with making movies: You're always going to make some stuff you believe is bad. This was mine.

## 2003

**ON** *S.W.A.T.*:

I loved *S.W.A.T.* In retrospect, I wish I could have had a bigger role in it, but I had a great time doing it, and it was a success. It was actually the coolest movie I've ever done, in terms of just a pure movie. It was the most entertaining and well done.

## 2004

**ON** *MINDHUNTERS*:

*MindHunters* was great because it was filmed around the time that I started getting in better shape. At that point, I was losing weight, really shaping up, really working on it, and I was able to do some great fight scenes in that movie, which brings back the whole Bruce Lee element. I got to live out that dream.

## 2005

**ON** *EDISON*:

First, I got to star with two of the greatest living actors in America, Morgan Freeman and Kevin Spacey. This was a completely intense role both mentally and emotionally for me. I had to be in the kind of condition needed to handle that. When I can work hard and get in shape and push myself physically, it makes me feel like I can do anything.

**Benefits achievable over the next 9 weeks (19 weeks since you started the Platinum Workout):**

The beginning outline of **SIX-PACK ABS**

Muscles **SO SCULPTED** you'll be dying to **HIT THE BEACH**

**DOUBLING** of **ENERGY LEVELS**

The **BEST PHYSICAL EXAM** stats of your life

**GREAT SHOULDER-TO-WAIST RATIO** producing a V-taper

phase three

# THE
# GOLD
# BODY

# TIME TO MUSCLE UP

**F**INALLY, **THE** preparations have been made. The fuse is lit. You're better conditioned and stronger now, ready to kick ass and take names. It's time to big up, baby.

For the next 4 weeks, en route to building muscle, torching body fat, and looking as diesel as an 18-wheeler, it's time for a traditional bodybuilding-style muscle-growth program. This is the most volume we've applied to individual body parts to date. Bombing my chest by doing multiple sets in rapid succession, for example, requires me to recruit more muscle fibers. And the more muscle fibers that are activated, the more potential there exists for growth. What's more, I experience a tremendous blood rush to the muscles, providing

**Man cannot remake himself without suffering, for he is both the marble and the sculptor.**

**—ALEXIS CARREL**

them with the nutrients they need to make me look toned—no, ripped. Every body part will be hit with some variation on that same theme for the next month.

As always, though, the Gold mix is alloyed into Platinum with some unexpected "specials" that make it unlike anything your body has ever experienced before. For example, exercises are often paired as supersets to keep your heart pumping while maximizing time efficiency. Over the course of an exercise, reps often rise and fall in steplike patterns for muscle stimulation and growth. One minute you're doing upper-body work and then we're sending you on a 40-minute run.

But the key to any muscle-building phase is the application of the progressive overload principle, which means that muscle tissue will only increase in strength and size when it's forced to handle more weight than it's handled before. Throughout this phase, always try to increase your weights while still hitting the target rep range. If the workout asks you to do 15 reps and you can do more, you're going too light. (Conversely, if you can't get to 15, you're going too heavy.) As the reps fall, train heavier still. And to keep the fat-burning fires stoked, Scooter mixes steady-state runs with inclines and intervals.

As you make your way through "Gold," bear one thing in mind: The pace of your initial gains will slow down. It happens inevitably to everyone, so don't be discouraged when it happens to you, too. It's like any sport: A guy picking up a basketball for the first time can probably double his skill set after a month of steady practice, but Carmelo Anthony's improvement would be imperceptible over 30 days. It's been a recurring theme of this book, but the human body is an amazingly responsive machine. As it adapts, further progress becomes that much harder to generate.

# Weeks 11 and 13: Muscle-Up Workouts (Weeks 12 and 14 follow)

- Warm up for 5 to 10 minutes using a treadmill, a stationary bike, or some other cardio apparatus before each workout. Jumping jacks or running in place will also do the trick.
- Select a weight that causes you to reach failure in the rep range given. This should be heavier in Week 13 than it is in Week 11.
- Any two exercises paired in supersets should be done back-to-back, without resting in between. Once you've finished the pair, rest 1 minute and

then do the additional sets. Also rest 1 minute when moving from one pairing to the next.

- Rest 1 minute between sets and exercises when doing straight sets.
- Complete the cardio workout outlined below.

## Monday

| EXERCISE | SETS | REPS |
|---|---|---|
| **Chest** *Superset:* | | |
| Barbell bench press | 2 | 15–20 |
| Pushup (feet elevated) | 2 | 15–20 |
| Incline dumbbell bench press | 1 | 15–20 |
| **Back** *Superset:* | | |
| One-arm dumbbell row | 2 | 15–20 |
| Bent-over barbell row | 2 | 15–20 |
| Pulldown | 1 | 15–20 |
| **Shoulders** *Superset:* | | |
| Upright row | 2 | 15–20 |
| Seated dumbbell press | 2 | 15–20 |
| **Scooter's ab circuit no. 3:*** | | |
| 1. Jackknife | 2 | 15–20 |
| 2. Hanging running man | 2 | 15–20 |
| 3. Crunch | 2 | 15–20 |

*Don't rest until you've done all three ab moves consecutively. Then rest 1 minute and repeat until you've done the required sets.

### Cardio:
1. Set the treadmill incline at 1.0 and find the speed that brings up your heart rate to 65 percent of maximum heart rate (MHR).
2. Increase your speed 0.5 every minute for the next 4 minutes.
3. Back off to your cruising speed for 2 minutes.
4. Continue alternating in this fashion until completing 30 minutes of total work.

# Tuesday

| EXERCISE | SETS | REPS |
|---|---|---|
| **Quads** *Superset:* | | |
| Barbell squat or leg press | 4 | 15, 20, 25, 10 |
| Leg extension | 4 | 10, 15, 15, 10 |
| **Hamstrings, glutes, and lower back** *Superset:* | | |
| Lying leg curl | 5 | 10, 8, 8, 6, 20 |
| Hyperextension | 5 | 10, 8, 8, 6, 20 |

# Wednesday

**Cardio:**
1. Set the treadmill incline at 1.0 and warm up for 5 minutes at 60 percent of MHR.
2. Raise the incline to 2.0 and run 1 minute at 80 to 85 percent of MHR.
3. Run 1 minute at 55 to 60 percent of MHR.
4. Continue alternating these two intervals for 20 minutes of total work.

# Thursday

| EXERCISE | SETS | REPS |
|---|---|---|
| **Arms** *Superset:* | | |
| Standing barbell curl | 5 | 10, 8, 6, 5, 20 |
| Dip (close grip) | 5 | 10, 8, 6, 5, 20 |
| *Superset:* | | |
| Preacher curl | 3 | 8, 8, 6 |
| Skull-crusher | 3 | 8, 8, 6 |

Repeat Monday's ab circuit.

# Friday

**Scooter's cardio circuit:**
1. Jump rope for 1 minute.
2. Without resting, do pushups for 30 seconds.
3. Without resting, jump rope for 30 seconds.
4. Without resting, do pushups for 30 seconds.
5. Rest 1 minute and repeat.
6. Continue in this fashion for 20 minutes of total work.

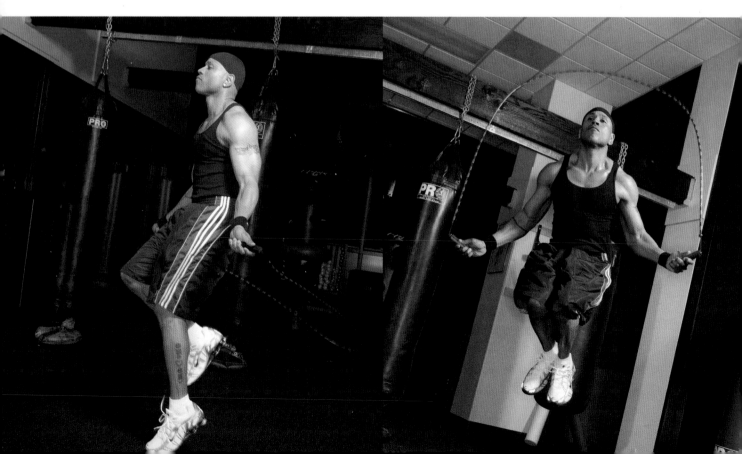

## FAST FOOD: THE FASTEST WAY TO GET FAT

Fast food is definitely fast; whether it's food is debatable. Many of the most popular offerings at fast-food restaurants contain 40 or even 50 ingredients. Hold up—last time I checked, chicken contained one ingredient: chicken. What's up with all that other stuff? Entire scientific labs are devoted to making fast-foodstuffs smell and taste better than they should with chemical flavorings, special odors, and a truckload of salt. How else could they make things like methylcellulose, potato starch, and autolyzed yeast extract taste like chicken? Add to these mystery ingredients a cup or two of cooking oil, butter, or margarine, and you've got a caloric gut-bomb that'll kick you clear off your nutritional track.

I know, you're saying: "But, LL, the stuff tastes so good! And I can just pick up a bucket of chicken on my way home from work." But I ask you: What price are you willing to pay for convenience? Are you willing to risk your health and the health of your family by "driving thru" to save a few minutes in the kitchen? I'm not, and my advice is to avoid the stuff altogether. I do understand that sometimes you'll be forced to do a drive-by eating, but in these circumstances you can choose alternative menu items to stay dialed in with your healthy eating plan. Call it damage control.

Because of customer demand and some seriously bad press (how many of you saw *Super Size Me*?), many restaurants nowadays offer healthier meal choices. Items such as salads with grilled chicken, steak, or fish; soups; baked potatoes; and yogurt with fruit are popping up in McDonald's, Wendy's, and Burger Kings around the country as viable alternatives to their regular fried fare. Other places offer customized menu options. Taco Bell, for instance, will replace the gooey sauce or cheese on an entrée with a mixture of tomatoes, onions, and cilantro when you order it "fresco," and at KFC you can actually order skinless, nonfried chicken breast. Not exactly soul food, but as close to a heart-friendly alternative as you're likely to find. Always ask for a fat-free salad dressing and use it sparingly, and request that your salad be prepared without cheese, that your potato be cooked dry, and that your burger be made with lettuce instead of that overprocessed bun. Restaurants can and will do these things for you, but they'll probably cop an attitude and take extra long to make it. But if you save yourself 10 to 15 grams of fat, it's worth the hatin' for a minute or two. As for regular, sugary soft drinks, just walk on by, as Dionne Warwick once said. If you have to have a pop, make it diet or skip it altogether and have water, lots and lots of water, to help dilute the huge sodium content of even the healthiest fast-food fare. More damage control.

Next, beware of the seemingly "healthy" juice, coffee, and drink bars around town. I mean, you'd think a smoothie would be better for you than a burger and fries, and in some ways it is—smoothies have very little fat. However, many are packed with calories, carbohydrates, and sugar. Have your smoothies made with water instead of sorbet or ice cream, and your coffee drinks made with fat-free milk and no whipped cream, and you'll be in good shape. If your coffee bar order has five adjectives, look out.

Most of all, educate yourself. Always check the nutritional content provided by the store either in house or on their Web site to see where you can subtract unneeded calories. Better yet, look up your favorite fast-food meal on the Internet for a reality check on their ingredients and nutritional content. Believe me, you'll think twice about ordering that again once you know what it contains.

Yes, fast food is easy, convenient, and cheap, but ultimately your health is paying the price, and I don't think any burger is worth that big of a hit.

(Sources: www.nal.usda.gov, www.bk.com, www.mcdonalds.com, www.tacobell.com, www.jambajuice.com, www.kfc.com)

## Saturday

| EXERCISE | SETS | REPS |
|---|---|---|
| **Upper body:** | | |
| Incline barbell bench press | 5 | 8, 8, 6, 15*, 6 |
| Pullup (assisted) | 5 | 8, 8, 6, 15*, 6 |
| Seated dumbbell press | 5 | 8, 8, 6, 15*, 6 |

*Drop set: Select a weight that causes you to fail at 5 reps. Lessen the weight and do 5 more reps. Lessen the weight again and do 5 more reps.

**Cardio:**

Run 40 minutes at 65 to 75 percent of MHR.

## Sunday

Active rest

# Weeks 12 and 14: Muscle-Building Workouts

- Warm up for 5 to 10 minutes using a treadmill, a stationary bike, or some other cardio apparatus before each workout. Jumping jacks or running in place will also do the trick.
- Each weight-training day's workout consists of four exercises targeting two body parts (except as noted on Friday).
- For the first and third exercise each day, do 5 reps, rest 15 to 20 seconds, and continue alternating until you've completed 20 reps. That's one set. Rest 2 minutes before going through the same progression again. Complete three such progressions.
- For the second and fourth exercise each day, do 3 reps, rest 15 to 20 seconds, and continue alter-

nating until you've completed 12 reps total. That's one set. Rest 2 minutes before going through the same progression again. Do three such progressions.

## Monday

**Chest:**
Incline barbell bench press
Barbell bench press
**Biceps:**
Standing barbell curl
Preacher or incline dumbbell curl
**Cardio:**
30 minutes on any apparatus at 65 to 70 percent of MHR.

## Tuesday

**Back:**
Bent-over barbell row
Seated cable row
**Triceps:**
Pushdown
Dip

## Wednesday

**Cardio: Scooter's sprint workout**
1. Warm up for 5 minutes at a casual pace (fast walk to slow run).
2. Set the treadmill incline at between 8 and 12 and run at 85 to 95 percent of MHR for 30 seconds.
3. Place your feet astride the treadmill and rest for 30 seconds.
4. Alternate for 15 minutes.
5. Lower the incline to 3.
6. Do another 15 minutes, but with the high intervals at 80 percent of MHR.

# Thursday

**Scooter's cardio circuit:**

1. Jump rope for 1 minute.
2. Without resting, do 30 seconds of pushups.
3. Without resting, jump rope for 30 seconds.
4. Without resting, do 30 seconds of pushups.
5. Rest 1 minute and repeat.
6. Continue alternating for 30 minutes of total work.

# Friday

**Shoulders:**
Seated dumbbell press
Upright row

**Abs:**
Machine crunch
Hanging running man
For abs, do 3 sets, 15 reps of each exercise in straight-sets fashion. Rest 30 seconds in between sets.

**Cardio:**

1. Set the treadmill at an incline of 10.
2. Walk uphill for 35 minutes at a speed of 3.5 to 4.5.

# Saturday

**Quads:**
Barbell squat, hack squat, or leg press
Leg extension

**Hamstrings:**
Lying leg curl
Romanian deadlift

# Sunday

Active rest

## THE PLATINUM SANDWICH

Forget peanut butter and jelly—the Platinum version is loaded with protein, provides some fiber, and packs a heck of a lot of vitamins and minerals.

Follow these instructions:

**1.** Start with 2 slices of whole-grain bread.

**2.** Grill or bake a chicken breast the size of a deck of cards.

**3.** Cook the chicken 3 to 5 minutes on each side, or until it's no longer pink on the inside. Place it on the bread.

**4.** Top with mustard and sliced tomato.

**5.** Add a side of mixed fruit and enjoy!

*Totals: 300 calories, 37 grams of carbohydrates, 33 grams of protein, 5 grams of fat*

—Christopher R. Mohr, PhD, RD

All these cartoon character MC's gettin' airborne
Takin' off like a hot air balloon
Goin' up up up, oh no kaboom

—LL Cool J, **"Mr. Smith,"** 1995

# RAP SESSION: BODY ETHICS

I alluded to this earlier in the Platinum Workout, but the beauty of this program is that it allows you to achieve the body you've always wanted without taking illegal and unethical—not to mention dangerous—shortcuts. I feel so strongly about this subject that this rap session features Ronald M. Green, PhD, the Eunice and Julian Cohen Professor for the Study of Ethics and Human Values, Dartmouth College. Dr. Green has also served as Director of the Office of Genome Ethics at the National Human Genome Research Institute of the National Institutes of Health.

**LL: We don't hear the word "ethics" spoken much anymore, so define it for us, Dr. Green.**

**Green:** Ethics concerns the way we should try to live our lives, both for our own self-fulfillment and as members of society. It's what's good or even best for us and others. It's based on the wisdom, thinking, and experience of generations of people. We think about and study ethics for guidance in how to make the choices that affect our lives and the lives of those we interact with.

**LL: Setting aside the medical and legal risks of steroids, isn't it important to accomplish things in life without looking for shortcuts?**

**Green:** I'm all for shortcuts. Why should I polish my car with a cloth when I can use an electric buffer? Why should I tough out a bad lung infection when I can take an antibiotic? But shortcuts are a bad idea when (1) they don't do the job right, (2) they're dangerous, (3) they force others to use them, and (4) no one is better off and everyone is worse off as a result.

Steroids pose at least three of these four problems: (1) They do the job—that is, they improve brute performance—in the short run, though not in the many ways that sound training does; (2) they wreak havoc with your health; (3) they force others, against their better judgment, to use them just to keep up and compete; and (4) in the end, if everyone does use them, no single athlete's position is improved, and yet everyone's situation is badly degraded.

A fifth consideration is that we want to keep sports genuinely interesting. If sports becomes a matter of how good your drug supplier is, it loses much of its interest. Winning's a big part of the game—but winning in ways that make the sport worth watching or participating in.

**LL: What do you say to young people who might see their heroes and role models accused of having taken performance-enhancing drugs and then think,** *If so-and-so can take them, why shouldn't I?* **After all,**

it seems to lead to great success by some objective measurements.

**Green:** It does. But these people are cheats. They knowingly break the rules to win. They may get the big prize if they conceal what they've done, but they haven't earned it fairly, and they're forever subject to exposure and humiliation, including loss of their honors. They deserve whatever bad things, from shame to sickness, come their way. It's a devil's bargain. Once you've made it, you're never free again. It means a life of lies.

**LL:** African Americans face some very specific health challenges, including higher risk for diabetes and high blood pressure. Yet young African Americans often don't have access to good nutritional information and healthy foods, compounding the problem. Do we as a society have an ethical imperative to address this and try to rectify it?

**Green:** Wouldn't it be terrific if the greatest African-American athletes, instead of ever being implicated in doping, became role models for good health and nutrition? There's lots of room here for them to do it. Young African-American men already smoke less than their Caucasian counterparts, I believe. That's the positive impact of sports in their communities. Athletics can play a major educational role in this instance.

**LL:** Peer pressure is especially intense among teens. If your friends are taking performance-enhancing drugs and pressuring you to experiment with them as well, how can you deal with this without either capitulating or being isolated from the group?

**Green:** I come back to the devil's bargain idea. Once you make that life choice, that ethical choice, you're never ever free of it. Even if you get out of a successful sports career with your health intact, you carry the risk of exposure and humiliation with you forever.

**LL:** Is gene doping the next huge issue in (presumably) illegal performance enhancement?

**Green:** Definitely. Gene interventions to alter muscle performance are already in development, and as of now they're virtually undetectable. So there will be a huge temptation for some athletes to cheat this way.

**LL:** Can it still be prevented or even managed, or is the genie out of the bottle?

**Green:** The genie is always out of the bottle. Where there's a will, there's a way. In all competitive enterprises, from sports to science, there will always be people who try to win big by breaking the rules. All we can do is (1) try to make it clear why we have the rules, (2) develop better ways of detecting cheaters, and (3) punish the hell out of them when they're caught. This all helps to reduce and minimize the problem. But it never eliminates it.

See what I mean I've changed I'm no longer A playboy on the run **I need something that's stronger** Friendship, trust, honor, respect, admiration This whole experience has been such a revelation It's taught me love and **how to be a real man** To always be considerate and do all I can

—LL Cool J, **"I Need Love,"** 1987

# chapter twelve

# THE PLAYER'S WORKOUT

IF YOU'VE survived this far, congratulations are in order. Pat yourself on the back. While you're at it, feel those traps getting bigger and thicker? Impressive, huh?

Now it's time for some fun and games, literally. The Player's Workout is a Scooter special. He explains: "I used to play dice in the park with the guys from a gym in Jamaica, Queens. Many of them were ex-cons who rolled the bones in the joint, know what I mean? When the numbers came up, we'd do that many pushups and pullups in the park. That's exactly how it went down. You can get an entire workout doing just that."

**I find that the harder I work the more luck I seem to have.**

**—THOMAS JEFFERSON**

1. Roll the die to get your exercise. Follow this guide: 6 numbers, 6 exercises:

   - 1 = pushup (regular version)
   - 2 = squat (body weight only)
   - 3 = mountain climber
   - 4 = situp or crunch
   - 5 = burpee with jump
   - 6 = lunge (alternating leg to leg)

## Week 15: The Player's Workout

The Player's Workout taxes your cardiovascular system while simultaneously building up your strength *and* muscle endurance. The only equipment you'll need is one die—and GUTS.

2. Roll it again to get your number of sets. What happens if you roll the same number on the second roll that you did on the first? You're in trouble, that's what. Give Scooter Pie 20 reps of each exercise consecutively without rest, and then continue.

If you're an adult and want to drink a little wine here and there, go for it. You don't have to live life like a stiff. Every now and then I'll drink some wine with dinner. Every now and then I'll be like, "Yo, give me a glass of wine"...I'll do that. This isn't about being perfect. This is about functioning at an optimum level while still enjoying your life.

But boozin' and *liquor* and all of that? Nah, I'm not down with that. That's not compatible with the Platinum Workout. And while alcohol does offer some benefits, other vices, such as cigarettes, do nothing but harm to your body. Of course, the biggest problem with most vices is that people turn to them initially for pleasure or a little stress reduction, only to become addicted when they can't stop.

Here's a rundown of major body vices, ranked in descending order from least harmful to most harmful. Beware of them all.

**Junk foods.** I've already covered this in the section on cheating, but it's worth addressing again because people who are addicted to junk foods such as chips, sodas, pizza, doughnuts, and sweets often treat them like a vice instead of a break from their diet. If you consume these foods compulsively, you're doing more than cheating; you're sabotaging your diet and the Platinum Workout program. You shouldn't eat junk food on more than 2 days a week, and even then you should do so in limited quantities. It's okay to have an occasional doughnut or slice of pizza as a way to take a break from your diet, but if you're craving these foods and then satisfying those cravings on a daily basis, you won't make the improvements you're capable of achieving.

**Alcohol.** Everybody knows that more than a little alcohol is harmful for your body, but many people try to rationalize drinking these beverages by claiming that they're healthy for your heart because they're high in antioxidants. Well, if you're drinking one glass of red or white wine per day, you may very well be doing your heart some good, but a lot of people don't stop there. If you're going to include more alcohol than this at a time, then you should get straight on what you're doing to yourself: You're taking a break from your Platinum Workout program to catch a buzz. That's okay if you do so infre-

quently. Just don't try to fool yourself into thinking you're doing something healthy for your body. Alcohol is a reactive chemical, and its effects in excess can be viewed as toxic. Alcohol is also very caloric (1 gram has 7 calories, making it far more caloric than the same quantity of carbs). It ain't the carbs in the beer that make you fat; it's the alcohol. My advice: Enjoy an occasional glass of wine or Courvoisier, but resist the temptation to crack open a few cold ones every time a game comes on the tube.

**Cigarettes.** What's the upside of smoking? Some say it's an effective way to reduce your weight. So is chopping off your arm, but that doesn't mean it's a good idea. Many people smoke because nicotine either reduces their perception of stress or increases their mental acuity. Nicotine by itself doesn't cause health problems—it's the smoke that does. But nicotine is highly addictive, meaning that you'll want to smoke more frequently. Of course, we know that smoking causes lung and other forms or cancer. It also causes respiratory problems and diseases (even if you haven't developed a disease, you almost certainly have some difficulty breathing if you're a heavy smoker). If you're a smoker, the one thing you can do to most improve your health, appearance, and longevity is to stop smoking. It's more important than improving your diet or exercising. Prioritize that ahead of killing yourself in the gym every day. Get off the lung darts—and then hit the gym.

**Drug abuse.** Every drug addict started as a recreational user. If you currently consider yourself a "recreational" drug user, then you're on one of two paths: Either you're going to grow up and stop using drugs altogether, or you're going to become an addict. It's virtually impossible to be a lifelong recreational drug user. My advice to you is to stop now while the choice is still in your hands. This is the worst of the vices because, in addition to the addictive nature of drugs and the health toll they take, they're also illegal. This is trouble that nobody needs. The bottom line on drugs is simple. If you're using, then you're not on the Platinum Workout program. Do yourself a favor and get completely off drugs before you even start to think about getting physically fit.

- Roll it again to arrive at the number of reps for each set. Here's where it gets a little tricky, though. (Let's hope you don't need a calculator.) Multiply the number that comes up on this third roll by the one that came up on the second roll. For example, if roll No. 2 was a 3, and roll No. 3 was a 4, multiply 3 × 4 to arrive at 12 reps.
- Rest 10 seconds between sets. Alternatively, do this workout with a fellow player and rest only as long as it takes him or her to rep out. First one out loses. You can make a lot of friends and enemies playing this game. Trust me.
- If you're really feeling like an animal, do a third Player's Workout this week using conventional dumbbell and barbell exercises instead of these body-weight moves. Use weights equaling 65 percent of your one-rep maximum.

# SCOOTER'S 1-MINUTE ABS TUTORIAL (OR, HOW TO LEAVE THE SADDLEBAGS BEHIND)

No body part presents more exercise options than your midsection. Part of the reason is that what people usually refer to as "abs" is actually four separate muscles: the rectus abdominis, the external obliques, the internal obliques, and the transverse abdominis. That's enough *CSI* jargon—suffice it to say that the latter three muscles run along the sides and kind of circle around the trunk and that the first, the rectus, is what we normally think of as the six-pack muscle. Note we said "muscle," not "muscles." The six-pack is actually one whole sheet of muscle crisscrossed by tendons that, when belly fat disappears, make it look like six individual itty-bitty muscles. The rectus abdominis makes you look good; the others are more functional; all of the above protect your lower back. So you want to hit all four for complete development.

The anatomy of the midsection has to be as complex as a space shuttle launch because so much human movement begins and ends there. It also explains why abdominal moves come in so many variations. At any one time, you'll see people crunching, raising their knees, twisting their midsections, or all of the above on the floor, on benches, using cable attachments, hanging from bars—you name it. Many gyms also house rows of machines dedicated to replicating those same moves with resistance. And we won't even get into all the contraptions you see being hawked on infomercials. Let's just say that a lot of it rhymes with *crunk*.

Follow these recommendations from Scooter in the context of your Platinum Workout, and you'll have rap-video abs like LL's in no time.

**1.** Vary your selection of abdominal exercises. Otherwise, your body will adapt to what you're doing and stop responding to the stimulus.

**2.** Your abdominals are like your other muscles. Don't train them every day. Plus, they're worked indirectly when you train most other body parts. Rest them. They need to recover.

**3.** As with most things in life, think quality, not quantity. I'll bet you cash money that if I force you to perform an abdominal move my way—the correct way—I can fry your midsection with 15 reps of almost any one exercise.

**4.** Train abs at the end of your workout. They'll be pre-exhausted from providing stability for other exercises, so when you finally train them, they'll get totally cooked.

**5.** Never pull on your neck with your hands when doing ab exercises. Your hands should almost cover your ears, as if someone is shouting at you. That'll prevent you from pulling.

**6.** Try to keep tension on your abs throughout the entire movement. If there's one training key to getting a six-pack like my man LL's, that's it: continuous tension throughout the entire move.

# HOW TO READ A FOOD LABEL

Successful dietary changes start with understanding how to read food labels. Without that basic knowledge, it's virtually impossible to help manage food intake and control energy balance.

The first thing to look at is serving size. If all the numbers listed are based on half a cup of the food in question, and you normally eat 2 cups' worth in a sitting, factor that into the equation. Having determined the proper serving size, check out the amount of calories in each serving. Then take a look at the fat content for each serving. In general, aim for foods that have 3 or fewer grams of fat for every 100 calories (aside from foods with healthy fats, such as mixed nuts and eggs). For example, if an item contains 300 calories per serving, it should provide fewer than 9 grams of fat per serving. Next,

within that total fat content, look at trans fat (see the example on the food label below). Ideally, this number should be zero. Trans fats provide no nutritional benefit whatsoever and actually can be harmful if consumed in high amounts.

Next, examine carbohydrate content, and under that umbrella term, keep an eye on the amount of sugar and fiber a product contains. Look for items that provide 3 or more grams of fiber and fewer than 10 grams of sugar per serving.

Finally, read the ingredient list. Generally, the fewer number of ingredients, the better. The ingredient listed first is the one that's most abundant in the product; the others follow in descending order of abundance. Look for items where sugar or one of its aliases, such as high-fructose corn syrup, isn't one of the first three ingredients on the list.

Check out the sample food label below for specifics on how to interpret different numbers.

—Christopher R. Mohr, PhD, RD

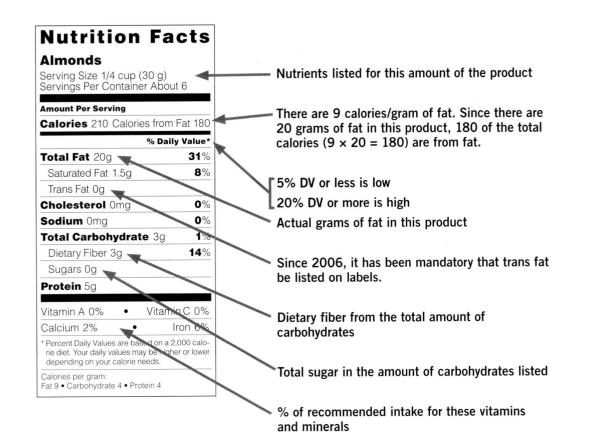

**Nutrition Facts**

**Almonds**

Serving Size 1/4 cup (30 g)
Servings Per Container About 6

**Amount Per Serving**

**Calories** 210  Calories from Fat 180

% Daily Value*

| | |
|---|---|
| **Total Fat** 20g | **31**% |
| Saturated Fat 1.5g | **8**% |
| Trans Fat 0g | |
| **Cholesterol** 0mg | **0**% |
| **Sodium** 0mg | **0**% |
| **Total Carbohydrate** 3g | 1% |
| Dietary Fiber 3g | **14**% |
| Sugars 0g | |
| **Protein** 5g | |

| | |
|---|---|
| Vitamin A 0% | Vitamin C 0% |
| Calcium 2% | Iron 0% |

* Percent Daily Values are based on a 2,000 calorie diet. Your daily values may be higher or lower depending on your calorie needs.

Calories per gram:
Fat 9 • Carbohydrate 4 • Protein 4

Nutrients listed for this amount of the product

There are 9 calories/gram of fat. Since there are 20 grams of fat in this product, 180 of the total calories (9 × 20 = 180) are from fat.

5% DV or less is low
20% DV or more is high
Actual grams of fat in this product

Since 2006, it has been mandatory that trans fat be listed on labels.

Dietary fiber from the total amount of carbohydrates

Total sugar in the amount of carbohydrates listed

% of recommended intake for these vitamins and minerals

# chapter thirteen

# KEEP DOIN' IT—

# BUILDING MUSCLE AND BURNING FAT

James Todd Smith, a.k.a. LL Cool J, has very good genetics, but he also has the conditioned mind of a professional athlete. He knows how to block out pain, and he knows how to focus on what he is doing. He's an entertainer, but I don't think the word *quit* is in his vocabulary. Whether he is filming a movie or doing dips with 150 pounds hanging from his waist, the focus is that of a Zen master. It's tunnel vision. He sees what he has to do. I guide him to the water. And then he takes the plunge.

—DAVE "SCOOTER" HONIG

**G**ET READY to take the plunge with me, because it's time for the second half of the Gold Phase. After developing your conditioning and strength endurance during the first 2 months of the program, you just finished a solid month of training devoted expressly to packing on size. Sorry if those broader shoulders, thicker arms, and smaller waist are starting to wreak havoc with your wardrobe. For our money, that's a small price to pay for those furtive glances being sent your way by the office receptionist.

Building on the progress you made during the first half of the Gold Phase, Scooter Pie integrates a lot of high-rep training (20-plus, going as high as 60) with classic muscle-growth schemes (8 to 10 reps) *and* pure strength training (6 or fewer reps) this month. This combination will bring an added component of muscular endurance—which you'll need for the Platinum Phase—while continuing to stimulate muscle growth and fat burning, which is our mantra.

Once again, the latest cutting-edge research coming out of universities is validating what Scooter has witnessed for decades working in the trenches with top-ranked boxers and other world-class athletes. Researchers in Japan started weight trainers on a 6-week muscle-growth program and then split them into two groups for further training: one that did strength training only and one that did mixed training, meaning strength training with the occasional 25-to-30-rep set thrown in for good measure. Lo and behold, the mixed training group continued gaining muscle mass, while the strength-only group actually gave a little muscle back. The startling finding, however, was that the mixed training group actually developed 5

percent more strength, measured by their one-rep max, during the second half of the experiment than the strength-only group did!

So what are you waiting for? Get a massage—and then get ready to throw down!

# Weeks 16 and 18: Super-Muscle-Building Workouts (Weeks 17 and 19 follow)

- Before each workout, warm up for 5 to 10 minutes using a treadmill, a stationary bike, or some other cardio apparatus. Jumping jacks or running in place will also do the trick.

## Monday

| MUSCLE GROUP | SETS | REPS | REST |
|---|---|---|---|
| Chest | 4 | 20–24 | 1½ minutes |
| Triceps | 3 | 25–30 | 1 minute |
| Back | 4 | 24–30 | 2 minutes |
| Hamstrings | 3 | 24–30 | 2 minutes |

Each set should combine two or three exercises. Use the repertoire you've already developed to combine exercises. (If you've forgotten, each exercise up to this point has been listed under the body part it works for easy reference.) For example, the first set for chest might be 10 reps of incline presses, followed by 8 reps of flat bench flies, and then 6 reps of weighted dips. Do whatever you want, as long as the numbers add up.

**LL'S FAT-LOSS TIP** Avoid cakes, cookies, pastries, and most other things you find sitting in vending machines. They're often loaded with trans fats and virtually devoid of useful nutrients, so steer clear.

You taught me if a task is once begun, Todd
# Never leave it 'til it's done, Todd
Be thy labor great or small, Todd
# Do it well or not at all

—LL Cool J, **"Big Mama (Unconditional Love),"** 2002

Continuing with the chest example, rest 1½ minutes and then repeat. Rest another 1½ minutes, and then repeat again. Rest another 1½ minutes, and then repeat again. Rest another 2 minutes and then go on to triceps.

## Tuesday

| MUSCLE GROUP | SETS | REPS | REST |
|---|---|---|---|
| Quads | 3 | 24–35 | 1½ minutes |
| Shoulders | 2 | 35–40 | 2 minutes |
| Biceps | 3 | 20–24 | 2 minutes |
| Calves | 3 | 40–50 | 2 minutes |
| Abs | 4 | 60–70 | 1 minutes |

## Wednesday

**Cardio:**
1. Warm up for 5 minutes at a casual place: slow walk/fast run.
2. Run 1 minute at 85 to 95 percent of maximum heart rate (MHR).
3. Run 1½ minutes at 55 to 60 percent MHR.
4. Continue alternating in that fashion for 40 minutes.

## Thursday

Active rest

## Friday

**Cardio:**
Run 45 minutes at 65 to 75 percent of MHR.

## Saturday

| MUSCLE GROUP | SETS | REPS | REST |
|---|---|---|---|
| Back | 4 | 8–10 | 1 minute |
| Chest | 4 | 8–10 | 1 minute |
| Triceps | 3 | 8–10 | 1 minute |
| Hamstrings | 4 | 8–10 | 1 minute |

Choose only one exercise per body part. Use compound movements, such as the bent-over row and bench press, for back and chest.

## Sunday

| MUSCLE GROUP | SETS | REPS | REST |
|---|---|---|---|
| Abs | 3 | 20 | 1 minute |
| Quads | 4 | 8–10 | 1 minute |
| Calves | 4 | 50 | 1 minute |
| Biceps | 3 | 8 | 1 minute |
| Shoulders | 4 | 8 | 1 minute |

Choose only one exercise per body part. Use compound movements, such as the squat for quads.

# Weeks 17 and 19: Super-Muscle-Building Workouts

## Monday

Rest

## Tuesday

**Cardio:**

1. Run uphill 150 yards.
2. Jog back to the starting line.
3. Repeat 5 times for six total hills runs.
4. Sprint a 440.
5. Jog a 440.
6. Alternate until completing four of each.

## Wednesday

| MUSCLE GROUP | SETS | REPS | REST |
|---|---|---|---|
| Chest | 6 | 5–7 | 1 minute |
| Triceps | 4 | 5–7 | 1 minute |
| Back | 6 | 5–7 | 1 minute |
| Hamstrings | 5 | 5–7 | 1 minute |

Choose two exercises per body part.

**Cardio:**

Run on a treadmill for 50 minutes at 65 to 70 percent of MHR.

## Thursday

Rest

# YOUR PRIMER ON PROTEIN

**1.** More than just your muscles are made from protein—so are your hair, nails, hormones, and enzymes, not to mention the antibodies that ward off sickness. All told, your body produces about 50,000 different kinds of proteins.

**2.** Uncle Sam, through the Recommended Dietary Allowances, recommends that you eat one-fourth of 1 gram of protein for every pound you weigh. This guideline was formulated during the 1940s and is about as backwards as that infamous "Dewey Defeats Truman" headline. If you're working out to build muscle and burn fat, you need about three times the government recommendation.

**3.** Spread your protein throughout the day. The human body can digest and process only so much protein, maybe 20 to 35 grams at one time. I weigh 210, which means I should be consuming 200 grams of protein a day, divided among six meals, rather than having, say, 90 percent at one sitting. Spacing it out is much better for muscle building, which in turn will help you with fat burning.

**4.** Milk, eggs, red meat, and fish are complete sources of protein, containing all eight of the so-called essential amino acids. Protein is also found in plant foods and elsewhere, but with the exception of soy, plant proteins are incomplete. In a vacuum, these collections of amino acids could not build muscle without augmentation.

**5.** Milk and other dairy products usually contain both whey and casein in varying amounts. For example, in cottage cheese, the curd is the casein, and the runny stuff between the curd is the whey. Milk, on the other hand, is 8 percent casein and 20 percent whey. The muscle set now prizes whey because it's so high in branched-chain amino acids.

**6.** Don't be afraid to drink protein shakes. I do. For one, it's inevitably easier to fill a blender with water and add powder than it is to cook a steak or chicken breast. And if you're abiding by the Platinum Workout's six-meals-a-day mantra, it's much easier to get down a liquid meal here and there than it is to eat nothing but whole foods all day.

Another advantage of shakes is digestibility. Your body can digest powders faster than animal tissues. This makes shakes particularly useful after a workout, during the recovery window. Finally, shakes are usually devoid of saturated fats, assuming you don't blend them with whole milk. (The one exception is weight-gain shakes, which have higher calorie counts than meal-replacement and protein shakes. Those usually contain saturated fats.)

# Friday

| MUSCLE GROUP | SETS | REPS | REST |
|---|---|---|---|
| Quads | 5 | 5–7 | 1 minute |
| Shoulders | 4 | 4–6 | 1 minute |
| Biceps | 4 | 6–8 | 1 minute |
| Calves | 3 | 15 | 1 minute |
| Abs | 4 | 30–40 | 1 minute 15 seconds |

**Cardio:**
Run on a treadmill for 50 minutes at 70 to 75 percent of MHR.

# DON'T (OVER)TRAIN IN VAIN

Overtraining is one of the biggest problems you're likely to encounter when you start a new exercise regimen. *Starting out, a lot of people are so gung ho that they go over the top, training to the point where they're actually tearing their bodies down, not building them up.* (Remember, you grow when you recover from training, not during your training!) While this type of overtraining is obvious, there's a more subtle, pervasive kind of overtraining that can build up gradually over weeks. If you're following the Platinum Workout program carefully, you may still run into problems with overtraining, and you'll need to back off a bit.

Here are some of the signs that you're overtrained—and some guidance on what to do about it—before it sends you down for the count:

## Symptoms of Overtraining:

**1. You're exhausted most of the time, but you have trouble sleeping at night.** This is one of the classic signs of overtraining—you just can't fall asleep, or you keep waking up, even though you feel like you need 10 hours of sleep every night. You may also notice that your body feels wiped out even when you're lying down.

**2. You're achy all over.** Beyond the specific fatigue and lactic acid you feel in your target muscles from individual training sessions, your body aches all over and you feel sluggish, almost like you've got a low-grade case of the flu.

**3. You're getting weaker.** When you first started your training program, you probably increased your reps and weights fairly quickly. Then you might have plateaued, no longer making dynamic progress. But if you're at a point where you seem to be dropping reps or the amount of weight you can use for a particular exercise, this may be due to overtraining. If it happens from one session to another, it's no big concern, but if you see a pattern of decreased strength, try backing off on your training rather than pushing harder.

**4. You're injuring yourself frequently in small ways.** If you find that you have a nagging or recurring pain in a body part that seems to show up even when you're not training it, this could be symptomatic of overtraining. In addition to the overtraining tips below, consider not training for this body part for a week or two.

**5. Your immune system is run-down.** If you're coming down with colds or other suppressed-immunity problems (cold sores, sties, etc.), this could be an indication that your training program is taxing your body too much, and your immune system is being overwhelmed.

## What to Do about Overtraining:

**1. Cut back on cardio.** Before you scrap your training program altogether, try cutting back just on your cardio, particularly on the intensity. Try 15 to 30 minutes of casual cardio, performed only about twice a week, where your heart rate rises only to an "active" level, not to its training level. This type of low-key cardio can actually help you recover from low-grade overtraining, while intense cardio can send you tumbling farther into the abyss of overtraining. Do this for 2 weeks before returning to your regular cardio training.

**2. Take 3 days off from training.** If you've been working out really hard, then you might see better gains by taking a break. (I know I keep saying it, but it's true: *You grow when you recover, not while you're training*.) You should only train hard with weights about 4 or 5 days a week. If you're doing more than this, then you'll ultimately end up overtrained.

**3. Eat more quality food.** Avid bodybuilders like to say that there's no such thing as overtraining; there's only undereating. The theory is that if you provide your body with more raw materials for recovery, you'll recover better and more quickly. If you're also on a strict diet regimen, you run the risk of sending yourself into an overtraining downward spiral fairly quickly. Try one or more of these nutrition quick fixes to help overcome low-grade overtraining.

- **Add more healthy fats:** Take flaxseed or fish oil, in either liquid or capsule form. Every day, add generous servings of olive oil, salmon, avocados, and nuts and seeds to your diet.
- **Bump up your complex carbs.** Eat a big healthy bowl of oatmeal every morning. Consume two pieces of whole-grain bread with your sandwich at lunch. Then, eat a large yam or generous serving of rice

(brown or white) with your dinner. Giving your body more complex carbs will help restock your muscle glycogen, the stored form of energy held in your muscle mass.

- **Add whole food protein.** Eat steak, chicken, eggs, cheese, and other forms of whole-food protein. These foods are more caloric than most protein shakes, but they're full of protein, nutrients, and beneficial fats.
- **Vary your diet and take a multivitamin/mineral:** It's possible that you may have a deficit in one or more specific nutrients. Often, people on a hard-core training and nutrition program limit their diets to so few foods that they end up cutting down on specific vitamins or minerals. Taking a multi and including more diet variety can help overcome this.

**4. Get a massage.** Massages not only feel good, but they're also good for your body, promoting the recovery and growth process. A weekly (or more frequent) massage can help you overcome overtraining and problem areas as well. In fact, I'm getting a massage as I write this sidebar.

**5. Soak in a hot tub or warm bath.** This is cheaper than massage, and it's also effective. Alternate warm baths with ice packs to stimulate blood flow to and away from problem areas. This "flushing" technique can help remove built-up toxins from an area of the body, allowing you to recover more quickly and overcome overtraining.

## LL Cool J: Built to Last

What were you doing in high school? LL Cool J was recording "I Need a Beat," the first-ever single released by Def Jam Records. Shortly thereafter, his first album, *Radio*, went platinum while earning major critical props as well. A legend was born.

That was a mere 16 years after James Todd Smith entered the world in Bayshore on New York's Long Island. His grandparents, mostly, raised him in Queens and North Babylon, and by 9, he was throwing down rhymes in his bedroom to the beats of the Sugar Hill Gang and others. Two years later, his grandfather handed him his first DJ system. Self-rechristened as LL Cool J, code for Ladies Love Cool James, he saw his first single, "Radio," drop 100,000 copies. Inspired by trailblazers such as Grandmaster Flash, Afrika Bambaataa, and the Treacherous Three, LL (along with Run DMC, Big Daddy Kane and Eric B and Rakim, and a select few others) gave birth to a new American art form, hip-hop, that has since reached the far corners of the globe.

LL's time on the charts has been off the charts by the standards of hip-hop, where acts often have a shorter shelf life than Chinese takeout. Twenty years have now passed and 20 million records have now been sold since the world heard LL rhyme sublime for the first time as he began his rapid climb into the prime time. Over those 2 decades, the résumé he has compiled is the kind of document that gets people feted at hall of fame ceremonies.

Just who is LL Cool J? He is a force of nature with a mike in hand, machine-gunning rhymes one moment, singing silky-smooth bedroom ballads like a modern-day Casanova the next. He has won three Grammy Awards. He has 12 platinum-selling albums to his name. He has turned tracksuits and a hat better suited for your grandfather—the Kangol—into iconic fashion symbols. He has starred in a hit TV show. He has acted in more than 20 feature films. He is the man whom every woman you know wants to meet.

He also displays that unlikeliest of rapper traits: modesty. "There were a lot of expansion franchises during that time, meaning there were record labels that were established," LL says in response to a question about why he made it when others didn't. "To extend the metaphor, I just happened to become part of the NBA as opposed to the ABA. God blessed me with this opportunity by putting me on the right team in the right

## SCOOTER'S *FAT-BURNING TIP*

Instead of walking forward for exercise, try walking backward on occasion—University of Oregon researchers found that it burns 25 percent more calories. If anyone looks at you funny, tell them Scooter says shifting into reverse increases your heart rate by nearly 50 percent and your oxygen use by more than 75 percent, compared with regular walking.

league at the right time." Yeah, and it doesn't hurt when you've got game like Dr. J.

If that's LL Cool J, who is Todd Smith? He is the devoted husband of 10 years to his own "Around the Way Girl," the former Simone Fenton, with whom he has four children: a son, Najee, 16; and three daughters: Italia, 15; Samaria, 10; and Nina, 5. He is a self-made intellectual who reads eclectically and voraciously in a home office that is essentially a library with a desk; who favors chess, not video games, in his rare moments of repose; and who displays something at least approaching a photographic memory when being interviewed. Nothing escapes him.

He is also an entrepreneur whose latest venture is an eponymous clothing line, for which he serves as a principal and, from all appearances, as a very hands-on comanager. As the namesake gives a guided tour of Todd Smith's Manhattan offices late one afternoon, his trademark merger of street and sophistication is on display everywhere, from the clusters of designers huddled around mannequins and drawings, to the racks of garments ready for sale at high-end department stores and boutiques, to what he himself is wearing: Yankees cap, Gucci sneakers, Seven jeans—only worn real baggy—

diamond earrings, wife beater underneath white dress shirt with French cuffs.

"This clothing company is just an extension of my spirit as well," Todd would say later that evening, inching across Manhattan during a rainstorm in the passenger seat of an SUV. "I just want to do great and interesting things with my life, God willing. Challenge myself, push myself, see how far I can take it. Oh, and it is challenging. Don't get it twisted. It is not easy. But I look at it like this, man. At the end of the day, whenever it's going to be over, it's going to be over anyway, so why not make the best of it? Why not make the most of it? Why not think as big as you possibly can? And then after you think as big as you possibly can, take actions to go in that direction. Why *not* do that? There's no reason not to—absolutely none."

Many of the line's garments—not to mention the office's front door—are emblazoned with a bold symbol with two spirals, interlocked. It stands for bravery and fearlessness, Todd Smith explains. When asked how involved he has been with the actual design of his line, the rap legend rolls up a pant leg, revealing the symbol tattooed on his own sculpted, muscular flesh. What do you think?

—JEFF O'CONNELL

You need to stay down, way down, because you're low down
Do that dance, the prince of rap is gonna throw down
Aiming to please while I'm killing emcees
I'm gonna keep on hitting you with rough LPs

—LL Cool J, **"Jack the Ripper," 1996**

Benefits available over 3 weeks (22 weeks since you started the Platinum Workout):

A **BODY** like **LL COOL J'S**

phase four
# THE
# PLATINUM
# BODY

# chapter fourteen

# TALES FROM THE RIPPED

**LL Cool J and "Scooter" Honig, overheard during one of their Platinum-level workouts:**

**Scooter:** The harder we work in the shorter amount of time, the more calories we burn. Even when he was doing those five reps, his heart rate was elevated.

**LL sprinting on a treadmill, breathing like a locomotive:** This is like somebody operating on you when you're awake. You gotta listen to this guy. It's like someone coming at you with a scalpel.

**Scooter:** Yo—

**LL:** No anesthesia. You're awake. **[Mock surgeon's voice]** "Uh-oh, we have bleeding." It's crazy.

**Scooter:** The only problem is, I don't bring him to the emergency room. He has to stay in the street. C'mon, we have 8 minutes left.

**LL:** Scooter, we had 8 minutes left 8 minutes ago.

**Scooter:** It's earl—

**LL:** Stop it. Stop it. Please. You're a bad actor. **[Steps off the treadmill and lets out a huge *Wheeeeeew!*]**

**Scooter:** He has a tendency to never get his heart rate on the machine. It's very weird. He's got no heart. I don't know what it is. Everywhere we go, every machine. You know what it is? He's got on these frickin' army boots. He doesn't have his running shoes on.

SO HERE it is, the moment you've been waiting for: the Platinum Phase. It's the wild-out with weights, know what I'm sayin'? This thing is a beast. For the next 3 weeks, cardio and weights will achieve equality, allowing you to achieve the ripped-to-the-bone, diamond-cut look that covers the front of this book. As always, this new phase is loaded with unexpected wrinkles designed to keep your body guessing and growing. Along with new weight workouts, including a full-body blast, we hit you with boxing workouts, wind sprints that will hammer your heart at 170 beats a minute, quarter-mile sequences wearing a weighted vest, and 40-minute distance runs. Change is good, know what I'm sayin'? After all, if you were the kind of person who accepted the status quo instead of reaching for the stars, you never would have picked up the Platinum Workout in the first place.

One new wrinkle you'll experience is supersets that pair weights with cardio blasts in the form of jumping rope. This is yet another Scooter special for building muscle while burning fat. It, too, is backed up by the latest research. Namely, scientists at the University of Missouri in Columbia were interested in comparing how fat burning during exercise and fat metabolism after exercise responded to one continuous 30-minute cardio session versus the same amount of work separated into three 10-minute blasts. In both instances, the subjects worked at 80 percent of their maximum heart rate, or MHR (an intensity you've already achieved in the Platinum Workout). Within the continuous session and the three separate sessions, fat burn in session was more or less the same. But when the subjects ate a fatty meal 12 hours after working out, those who had staggered their cardio showed significantly less fat in their bloodstream.

At the end of the 20th week, Scoots hits you with a workout consisting of moves performed one arm or leg at a time. As always, science gives method to the madness of King Scooter. For one, this will mercilessly reveal any strength imbalances existing between the left and right sides of your body. This training style also will require your body to correct those imbalances, since your strong side will no longer be allowed to cover for its weaker half.

That's not all, though. Training one arm or leg at a time also allows you to work your core muscles at the same time. Scientists from the Memorial University of Newfoundland (St. John's) tested the activation of core muscles (upper lumbar muscles, spinal erectors, and lower abdominals) in subjects doing chest presses and shoulder presses one arm at a time versus two arms at a time. They found that lifting one arm or leg at a time dramatically increased core activation—in the case of the bench press, by as much as 300 percent more for lower abs.

To make this final phase really crazy and hyped up, Scooter and I are asking you to use a technique that has been one of my most closely guarded secrets for years. At certain points in the workout, we're going to ask you to hold a weight in the position of full contraction for several seconds, rather than returning it immediately to the start position without pause. Hard-core workout guys have used this technique for years because they've known intuitively that it really fries their muscles, and recent research confirms that it works. Exercise scientists at the University of Connecticut at Storrs had 14 track-and-field athletes do three 3-second "holds" on the leg press before working the machine for another 30 seconds. Their leg-press strength increased by 6 percent when they preceded the longer set with the isometric contractions.

You'll also be doing your most intense cardio over the next 2 weeks. At times, you'll feel like you have a speed bag in your chest and Ali's messin' with it. *So be forewarned: This phase is not easy.* Even though I'm used to it, I still have to build up to it. Doing heavy inclines and then heavy pullups when your heart rate is so *high* going *in*? It's like sitting down to Thanksgiving dinner completely full—dessert, coffee, sambuca: everything. *Then* you sit down to eat. That's what doing heavy weights and then getting on a treadmill is like. It's like stuffing cardio into a body that's almost maxed out in terms of heart rate already. Makes it *very* difficult. It's *crazy.* It's nuts. It's the most exhausting, it's the most terrifying, it's the most painful yet rewarding part of my life. That's why I do it, and you can, too. It's the same reason people run marathons and climb mountains. There's something about reaching the summit and planting your flag that takes your whole life to another level because you believe in yourself.

That's what this phase is about: peaking. I don't stay in the Platinum Phase all the time; I dip back down to other phases. I'm being totally honest about it. It's ridiculous, but you got to do it if you want it. It's a thing inside, man. It's mountain climbing. And once you get there, it's the most amazing and exhilarating feeling in the world. Seriously.

So can you handle it? Let's find out.

# Week 20: LL's Most Hard-Core Workouts

- Before each workout, warm up for 5 to 10 minutes using a treadmill, a stationary bike, or some other cardio apparatus. Jumping jacks or running in place will also do the trick.

- When doing one of Scooter's circuits, don't rest in between sets until you finish the last move. Then rest 1½ minutes, except as noted. Repeat the circuit until you've completed the number indicated under "sets."
- When doing straight sets, rest 1 minute between sets and exercises, except as noted.

## Monday

| EXERCISE | SETS | REPS |
|---|---|---|
| **Chest, biceps, and cardio** | | |
| *Scooter's chest/cardio circuit No. 1:* | | |
| 1. Incline barbell bench press | 2 | 10–12* |
| 2. Incline pushup with tubing | 2 | 10–12* |
| 3. Jump rope | 2 | 2 minutes at 90 percent of MHR |
| *Scooter's chest/cardio circuit No. 2:* | | |
| 1. Barbell bench press | 2 | 10–12* |
| 2. Incline dumbbell fly | 2 | 10 |
| 3. Treadmill run | 2 | 2 minutes, 3 incline, 90 percent of MHR |
| 4. Weighted dip | 2 | 10–12* |
| 5. Boxing drills | 1 | 2 minutes at 90 percent of MHR |
| Rest 1 minute. | | |
| *Scooter's biceps/cardio circuit:* | | |
| 1. Standing barbell curl | 3 | 4–6 |
| 2. Incline dumbbell curl | 3 | 8–10 |
| 3. Preacher curl | 3 | 12–15 |
| 4. Sprinting with tubing | 3 | 1 minute at 90 percent of MHR |

*Hold the 5th or 6th rep in the most difficult position for 5 seconds before continuing.

# RAP SESSION: FEATS OF FEET

Along with being one of the world's leading cardio experts, Paul D. Thompson, MD, is director of the preventive cardiology program and of cardiovascular research at Hartford Hospital in Connecticut and professor of medicine at the University of Connecticut in Farmington. Dr. Thompson has been an author of more than 140 scientific articles on topics including the effects of exercise training on preventing and treating heart disease, the risk of sudden death during exercise, and the effects of exercise on lipid metabolism. These research efforts have been supported by grants from the American Heart Association; the National Heart, Lung, and Blood Institute; and the National Institute of Child Health and Human Development. He is a past president of the American College of Sports Medicine.

**LL: Dr. Thompson, what's the single most important reason someone should be doing cardio?**

**Thompson:** To maintain their exercise capacity as they grow older. In other words, to maintain their ability to perform the tasks of daily living and more difficult tasks as they age. It also reduces the risk of cardiovascular disease by helping to control body weight and blood pressure. In myriad ways it improves the quality of your life.

**LL: Give me a frame of reference: All things being equal, is doing cardio going to add 2 years or 20 years to my life?**

**Thompson:** Of the two, I think it would be much closer to 2 years. But it has less to do with the length of one's life than the quality of one's life.

**LL: When we hear about an experienced runner like Jim Fixx just keeling over in the street—should we be worried about that?**

**Thompson:** You should at least know about it. You shouldn't ignore symptoms that come on with exercise and go away with rest. Even someone who's in reasonably good shape can have underlying heart disease that can cause a sudden cardiac death. There are people who have things come out of the blue. You should be aware of it, you should pay attention to your symptoms, and you shouldn't think that exercise is a panacea.

**LL: In the aftermath of the Human Genome Project especially, pharmaceutical companies are finding that responses to drugs are often highly individualized based on genetics. Is it possible that cardio prescription will become similarly individualized?**

**Thompson:** That's already been found. We've reported on one gene that affects exercise performance, and another research group has found another. It's probably going to be much more complex than finding a single gene, but there's no doubt at all that these factors can affect exercise performance. Your response to exercise training is almost certainly going to have a genetic component.

**LL: What's the most exciting avenue of research in cardiovascular exercise right now?**

**Thompson:** I think it's that interaction of genetic factors and exercise performance that you just brought up. Finding genes that are associated with superior performance. It's going to be *much* harder than people think, but it will be very interesting. Another fascinating avenue of research is why people age at different rates. That will be increasingly important.

**LL: What are you studying at present?**

**Thompson:** We're interested in why exercise can hurt skeletal muscles in people taking cholesterol-lowering medications such as statins. In rare instances those drugs can cause muscle problems, and the problems seem to be more common in people who exercise. We're interested in what the molecular changes are that cause this sort of response.

**LL: What have you learned?**

**Thompson:** We're in the early stages of our research, but when we do muscle biopsies on subjects after they've exercised on and off statins, we've been able to show that there are indeed changes in the genes and how they're expressed in the muscle.

**LL: With all this great new research being made available, why are people still getting fatter and fatter?**

**Thompson:** We're genetically endowed to hunt and gather food, but when we're not doing that, we save energy. That was how we survived at one time in history; we didn't waste energy. So it's hard to convince people in this society to waste energy when genetically they're engineered not to.

# Tuesday

### Cardio:

Run on a treadmill or other cardio machine for 40 minutes at 75 percent of MHR.

# Wednesday

| EXERCISE | SETS | REPS |
|---|---|---|
| **Total-body training:** | | |
| 1. Pullup (weighted) | 4 | 5–7, 5–7, 10, 12–15 |
| 2. Barbell squat | 4 | 5–7, 5–7, 10, 12–15 |
| 3. Seated barbell press | 4 | 5–7, 5–7, 10, 12–15 |
| 4. Deadlift | 3 | 5–7, 5–7, 10 |
| 5. Skull-crusher | 3 | 5–7, 10, 12–15 |

Rest 2 minutes between sets and exercises for this workout.

# Thursday

Rest

# Friday

### Scooter's track circuit:

1. Run 440 meters (equals once around track).
2. Rest 30 seconds.
3. Sprint 100 yards.
4. Walk the turn.
5. Do 30 seconds of rapid-fire pushups.
6. Sprint 100 yards.
7. Run an 880 as fast as you can.
8. Jog a 440.
9. Rest 3 minutes.
10. Repeat as many times as possible without working more than 35 minutes.

# Saturday

Rest

# Sunday

| EXERCISE | SETS | REPS |
|---|---|---|
| **Legs, lower back:** | | |
| Unilateral leg press | 4 | 8–10 |
| Unilateral leg extension | 2 | 8–10 |
| Unilateral leg curl | 4 | 8–10 |
| Hyperextension | 3 | 5 |

### Cardio:

1. Warm up for 5 minutes at a casual (a slow walk to a fast run) pace on a treadmill.
2. Jog 1 minute at 50 to 55 percent of MHR.
3. Sprint 1 minute at 90 to 95 percent of MHR.
4. Continue alternating in this fashion for 30 minutes of total work.

# Week 21: LL's Most Hard-Core Workouts

- Before each workout, warm up for 5 to 10 minutes using a treadmill, a stationary bike, or some other cardio apparatus. Jumping jacks or running in place will also do the trick.
- When doing one of Scooter's circuits or supersets, don't rest in between sets until you finish the last move. Then rest 1½ minutes, except as noted. Repeat the circuit until you've completed the number indicated under "sets."
- When doing straight sets, rest 1 minute between sets and exercises, except as noted.

# Monday

### Cardio:

Run 30 minutes at 70 to 75 percent of MHR.

# Tuesday

| EXERCISE | SETS | REPS |
|---|---|---|
| **Scooter's back/cardio circuit:** | | |
| 1. Pulldown | 5 | 5, 7, 10, 12, 15 |
| 2. Bent-over barbell row | 5 | 5, 7, 10, 12, 15 |
| 3. Seated cable row | 5 | 20 |
| 4. Box jump | 5 | 1 minute |
| **Triceps, legs:** | | |
| Pushdown | 2 | 6, 8, 10 |
| Skull-crusher | 2 | 6, 8, 10 |
| Dumbbell pulse squat | 2 | 3 minutes* |

*Alternate 20 seconds of fast squatting with 10 seconds of rest.

# Wednesday

| EXERCISE | SETS | REPS |
|---|---|---|
| **Scooter's shoulders/ cardio circuit:** | | |
| 1. Seated dumbbell press | 5 | 5 |
| 2. Bent-over lateral raise | 5 | 8–10 |
| 3. Upright row | 5 | 5 |
| 4. Jump rope | 5 | 1 minute |
| 5. Explosive pushup | 5 | 30 seconds |

# Thursday

**Cardio:**
  1. Warm up for 5 minutes at a casual (a slow walk to a fast run) pace on a treadmill.
  2. Jog 1 minute at 50 to 55 percent of MHR.
  3. Sprint 1 minute at 90 to 95 percent of MHR.
  4. Continue alternating for 30 minutes.

# Friday

Rest

# Saturday

| EXERCISE | SETS | REPS |
|---|---|---|
| **Scooter's leg superset:** | | |
| 1. Squat | 3 | 15–21* |
| 2. Leg extension | 3 | 15–21* |
| **Scooter's leg superset:** | | |
| 1. Lying leg curl | 4 | 10 |
| 2. Romanian deadlift | 4 | 10 |
| **Biceps:** | | |
| Standing barbell curl | 2 | 15† |
| **Scooter's biceps superset:** | | |
| 1. Preacher curl | 1 | 20‡ |
| 2. Incline dumbbell curl | 1 | 20‡ |

*Select a weight that causes you to fail at 5 to 7 reps. Reduce the poundage and do the reps remaining till your 15th to 21st.

†Stop and reduce poundage once during set.

‡Stop and reduce poundage twice during set.

# Sunday

MORNING

| EXERCISE | SETS | REPS |
|---|---|---|
| **Scooter's chest/back/ cardio circuit No. 1:** | | |
| Incline barbell bench press | 4 | 10 |
| Pullup | 4 | 10 |
| Boxing drills | 4 | 2 minutes |
| **Scooter's chest/back/ cardio circuit No. 2:** | | |
| Dumbbell bench press | 4 | 10 |
| One-arm dumbbell row | 4 | 10 |
| Jump rope | 4 | 1 minute |
| Stepup | 4 | 1 minute |

**Cardio:**

1. Jump rope for 1 minute at a pace equal to 100 to 150 rope turns.
2. Rest 45 seconds.
3. Continue alternating in this fashion for 20 minutes.

EVENING:

**Track workout:**

1. Run a 440 in 1:15 to 1:30 minutes.
2. Do 1 minute of pushups.
3. Do 1 minute of squat thrusts.
4. Rest 1 minute.
5. Jump rope a 440.
6. Rest 1 minute.
7. Repeat 1–6 two more times.
8. Rest 1 minute.
9. Run an 880 as fast as you can.
10. Jog a 440.
11. Rest 30 seconds.
12. Do five 100-yard sprints, jogging back each time.
13. Rest 1 minute.
14. Repeat numbers 8 to 13 one time.

# LL COOL J'S LIFE INSURANCE POLICY

Pilots sitting in their cockpits confront so many dials and gauges, you might think they also needed to be rocket scientists to fly. No doubt all that information plays a pivotal role in safe flight, but you can bet that one or two of them—say, altitude and engine temperature—get eyeballed particularly closely and often.

The same goes for your body. A nearly infinite number of measurements can be taken, but if I had to single out one that you should really keep an eye on, it's your blood pressure. What is it? Well, when your heart pumps, the liquid in question is blood. Blood pressure refers to the amount of blood produced by that pumping action and the resistance that blood encounters as it flows throughout your body. Many health professionals argue that this is the single most important diagnostic indicator of long-term health.

While normal blood pressure is considered to be 135/85 mm Hg, optimal is considered 115/70. If your blood pressure is lower, you'll think more clearly, steer clear of strokes that could paralyze you, keep your veins and arteries pumping away, and live longer. Pretty good deal all around, huh?

The first line of defense against elevated blood pressure is lifestyle, including diet, exercise, and stress management. For one, avoid consuming excessive salt (a.k.a. sodium), as it can temporarily elevate blood pressure. Also, eat plenty of fruits and vegetables, maintain your ideal body weight, exercise according to Scooter's workout designs, and don't booze it up. If these lifestyle changes alone don't normalize your blood pressure, at some point your doctor may prescribe medication. Diuretics help rid your body of excess sodium. Beta-blockers decrease the squeezing function of the heart. ACE inhibitors lessen the internal resistance to blood flows.

Another key "cockpit gauge" is cholesterol. Cholesterol and blood pressure are independent of each other, but if someone has elevated cholesterol for a long period of time, their arteries can harden, which in turn can raise blood pressure. Arteries harden when fatty substances deposit along their walls, leading to plaque formation. When the blockages created by this plaque buildup become severe enough, they can lead to heart attacks and strokes. The latter are basically heart attacks in the brain.

Cholesterol is actually part of a bigger picture called your lipid profile. First, you've got high-density lipoproteins (HDL), often called good cholesterol because it scavenges around the walls of your cardiovascular system, bringing the other kind of cholesterol back to the liver. (Let's call that good scavenger stuff "catfish" cholesterol.) What it scavenges is low-density lipoproteins (LDL), the so-called bad cholesterol. (Let's call that "sticky" cholesterol.) Then there are triglycerides, or blood-circulating fats. Those numbers are extremely important individually, but the ratios between and among them can be equally important. The latest research shows that extremely aggressive lowering of LDL to below 70 with the use of statin drugs can not only halt progression of arterial plaque but also reverse it. Also, the Framingham (Massachusetts) Heart Study data showed that low HDL may be a better predictor of increased cardiovascular risk than elevated LDL is.

A number of factors contribute to your personal lipid profile. Some you can control; others you can't control as easily. But you've got to work on it.

"Medical doctors really look at blood pressure, cholesterol, family history, and smoking," says Robert S. Palazzo, MD, FACSM, an attending cardio-thoracic surgeon at the North Shore Long Island Jewish Health System. "Those are the key things. If you're a nonsmoker, if you don't have any family history, if you've got good cholesterol, and if you've got good blood pressure, then the likelihood that

you're going to have significant coronary disease is very low for now."

Dr. Palazzo emphasizes that genetics plays a major role in blood pressure and cholesterol. Don't use what you think you know about your genes as a crutch, though. Genetics plays a role in learning how to dance, but lessons help.

*Not* having a worrisome family history hardly means that you're off the hook. "Some people without a family history of coronary disease develop it nonetheless," says Dr. Palazzo. "And why do they do that? Usually because they have bad habits like smoking."

If this all sounds a bit scary, here's the good news. "Along with dietary changes, exercise helps keep good cholesterol high and bad cholesterol low," says Dr. Palazzo. "Cardiovascular exercise and weight training—especially a cardio workout with weights, the way Scooter does it—also both promote weight loss, which is preventive of diabetes, another huge risk factor for heart disease."

After the age of 35, check your blood pressure, cholesterol levels, and heart rate every 6 months to a year. While elevated numbers can be problematic, an even more telling indicator may be the changes in these numbers. You won't recognize changes if you don't know your personal baseline. So start keeping track.

# chapter fifteen

# YOU MADE IT!

**The reward of a thing well done is to have done it.**

**—RALPH WALDO EMERSON**

**D**URING THE final week of the Platinum Workout, LL and Scooter insist that you do—drum roll, please—absolutely nothing? Straight up.

By getting this far in the program, you've accomplished something that you have every right to be proud of. So take some time to hang out with your friends, go shopping for some new clothes—better yet, reward yourself with a massage. Spend your week enjoying how good you look and showing off your new body.

To that end . . .

## Week 22

Do nothing. It's a wrap.

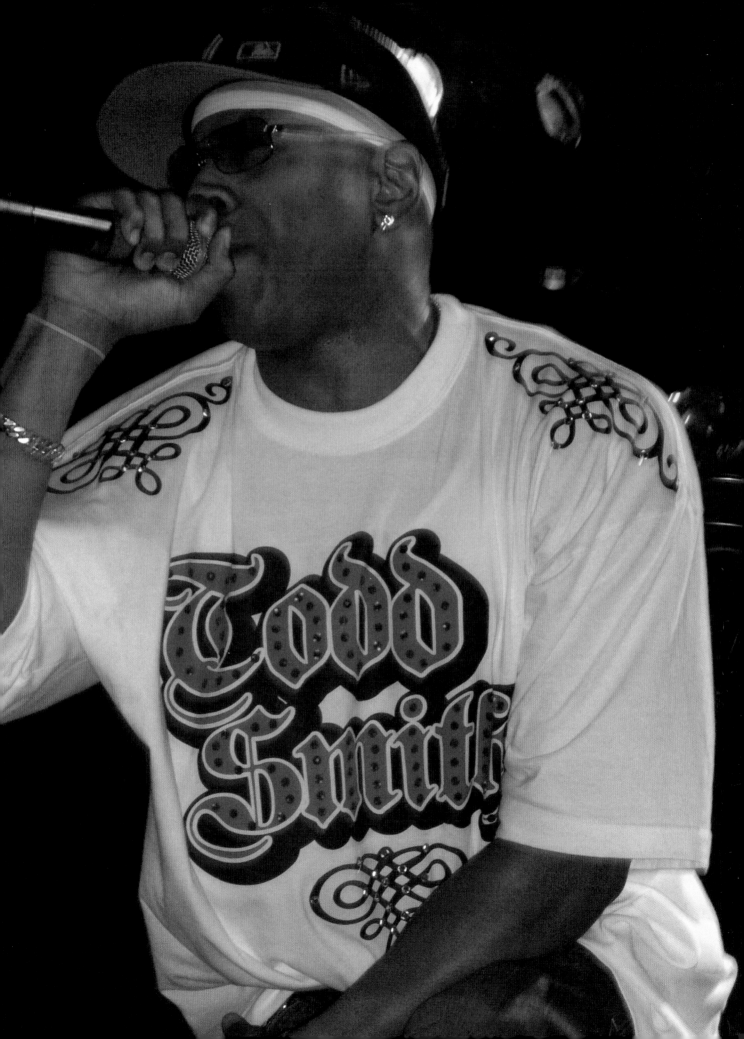

# 9 REASONS YOU'RE NOT LOSING WEIGHT

I'm used to pushing it to the outer limits when recording new joints, but losing body fat to shape up isn't an exercise in extremes; it's a matter of balance. Do too much or too little of one thing and you may not lose body fat as quickly as you expect. To achieve the best results, practice the discipline of moderation. If you're not seeing the results you want, consider that the reason may be one of the following, and use my personal quick fix to correct the problem in short order.

**1. You're adding muscle mass faster than you're losing body fat.** This is a best-case scenario—your program is working, but you just aren't recognizing it. If the scales are giving you bad news, it could be because you're increasing your muscle mass faster than you're losing body fat. Muscle mass is heavier than body fat, and when your body starts to make this shift, it adds muscle mass more quickly than it sheds body fat. **LL's quick fix:** All you need in this case is an attitude adjustment. Use your mirror, pay attention to how your clothes are fitting, and take the compliments you receive to heart. They're all much better gauges of your success than a number on a scale. If everything seems to be pointing to success except the needle, ignore it.

**2. You're eating too much.** If you're committing this sin, you probably know it without my telling you more about it. If you're going to lose body fat, you have to be in a calorie deficit. There's a limit to how many calories you can burn by exercising each day, so you have to limit caloric intake to make sure

you're in a deficit. **LL's quick fix:** One thing you may have noticed when you started this program is that your appetite increased. Channel that into opportunity: Emphasize healthy low-calorie foods such as vegetables and lean protein sources so that you can still consume a large volume of food without stuffing yourself full of unwanted calories. Satiety (that satisfied feeling from eating) can be achieved with fewer calories when you eat crunchy, low-calorie foods such as vegetables.

**3. You're not eating enough.** "Enough" in this case may mean that you're not eating enough calories, you're not eating often enough, or both. If you habitually eat only a large meal or two a day, you may be undereating. Strangely, this can allow calories to be stored as body fat. When you eat a large quantity of food in a sitting and then neglect to eat for hours on end, your body tends to hoard the calories it doesn't need from these infrequent meals as body fat. **LL's quick fix:** To find success, eat fewer calories in a sitting, and eat more frequently. This may mean actually increasing the total number of calories you consume a day, but your body will be more inclined to burn them than to store them as body fat. Strive to take in up to six meals a day, distributing the number of calories you consume fairly equally from one meal to the next.

**4. You're not training enough.** If you're following the program as I've laid it out, you're training enough. The only suggestion I can offer is to train with more intensity. If you're not keeping up, but you're doing what you can, then just keep going at your pace. Your results will come. On the other hand, if you're skipping workouts because you're busy or because you don't feel like it, you're just not going to achieve results that are as impressive as you want. **LL's quick fix:** The first thing you have to realize is that you do have time to work out. Get in 15 minutes here and there each day. Make the commitment. That's when you'll see real results.

**5. You're training too much.** This may be a shocker, but training too much, too hard, or both can undermine progress. Keep in mind that the workouts themselves tear down your body. You make progress and grow after training, during recovery. **LL's quick fix:** If you are overtraining (see "Don't [Over]Train in Vain" on page 190 for more on this), you may need to back off on your training volume or frequency. You should limit weight training to about 4 days a week, and you should include at least 1— if not 2—full rest days each week.

**6. You're not performing enough cardio.** When you're weight training, you're jacking up your metabolic rate by encouraging calorie burning and adding muscle mass. Cardiovascular training (walking, jogging, running, or using any of the gym machines such as treadmills, bicycles, or stairclimbers) is also important for burning calories and ultimately for burning body fat. **LL's quick fix:** Make sure that you perform as much cardio as the program prescribes.

**7. You're performing too much cardio.** Many people think they can climb onto a treadmill and just keep moving until their body is perfect. That's not the case. Performing an excess of cardio (either in intensity, frequency, or duration) can take your body over the edge into a state of overtraining, and it can burn muscle mass rather than body fat. Either way, your cardio actually can end up working against your goal of shedding body fat and adding lean muscle mass. **LL's quick fix:** If you think this is the case, cut back on your cardio somewhat—either the length of sessions, the frequency, the intensity, or a combination of these variables.

**8. You're eating too many carbs.** If you consume a high percentage of your calories from carbohydrates, you may be impeding your ability to shed body fat— and you may not be encouraging enough muscle growth if you're simultaneously not eating enough protein. Carbs, especially sugary or starchy carbs, can make you feel sluggish and negatively affect your blood sugar. They can also encourage you to store body fat. **LL's quick fix:** To avoid this problem, cut back on carbs in general, relying more on slow-burning sources such as oatmeal, brown rice, and yams, which have a less negative impact on your blood sugar levels. Particularly avoid consuming sugary and starchy carbs by themselves. These include sodas, pasta, white bread, and candy.

**9. You're not eating enough carbs (before and after you work out).** Nutrition is complex and specific to each individual. You need to cut back on sugary carbs in general, but you want to include them before and after your workouts, when they will help drive nutrients into your cells. Pre- and post-workout, they deliver nutrients to your muscles, stimulated by your workouts, rather than to your body-fat stores. **LL's quick fix:** Consume as many as 50 grams of simple carbs in the half hour both before and after you work out. (Check labels to see how large of a portion this equates to.)

Benefits achievable over the next 4 weeks:

A tighter butt, firmer thighs—and **NO MORE CHICKEN ARMS**

**METABOLISM** like a **FAT-BURNING FURNACE**

Your best body ever **4 WEEKS FROM NOW!**

hase five (for women)

# THE DIAMOND BODY

# chapter sixteen
# GETTING CUT AND SPARKLING

**D**IAMONDS ARE forever. Kanye West and James Bond both said that, so you know it must be true.

Scooter and I both feel strongly that women should train like men, and vice versa. The fear held by some of you ladies—namely, that lifting weights will bulk you up, even make you look like a man—doesn't hold water. Think of it this way: Most of the guys in your gym *want* to look big, ripped, and jacked, right? That's why they're there. Yet the majority can't achieve that look by pushing iron—and they've got testosterone coursing through their veins naturally! (Things will be different once they do the Platinum Workout, though.) As a woman, you really shouldn't waste a second worrying about morphing into a muscle

man. (Believe me, ladies, I want to be the hardest thing in the bed.) In fact, weights are just what the doctor ordered if you want toned, sculpted muscles of the kind guys everywhere find sexy, yours truly included. After all, carbon only turns into a diamond after pressure is applied.

To check ourselves, however, we consulted with David R. Pearson, PhD, CSCS, an associate professor of physical education and director of the Strength Research Laboratory at Ball State University in Muncie, Indiana, as well as a member of the *Men's Health* magazine editorial advisory board. Dr. Pearson gave us his take on how differently men and women should train, if at all. Specifically, he told us, "There are differences in how men and women respond to strength training, but at the same time, there isn't any reason men and women should train differently."

Precisely. Score one for Scooter Pie and me. Dr. Pearson went on to emphasize that women simply don't bulk up like men do, and with good reason. "There seems to be something inherently different in the sexes in how their bodies respond to stress [from resistance exercise]," he explained. "Women, for the most part, get stronger without increasing muscle mass to a pronounced degree. Men, on the other hand, respond by increasing muscle mass. The most obvious explanation for that difference is hormonal, but that doesn't completely explain why women can continue to get stronger without an appreciable increase in muscle mass and why at some point in their training, men's muscle shifts from a recruitment phenomenon to an enlargement phenomenon. Hormones are hugely important, but all of the questions have yet to be resolved."

All of which brings us to the Diamond Workout plan, which has been designed especially for women, emphasizing butt, hamstrings, and other body parts that we know you want to firm up (although the Diamond program is certainly difficult enough to tax most men). We pulled out all the stops on this one—Scooter and I rolled up our sleeves and collaborated directly with the Platinum Workout exercise consultant, Jimmy Peña, fitness director of *Muscle & Fitness* magazine and one of the nation's most dynamic young fitness professionals. The net result is a radical 4-week shape-up program for women that is nothing short of amazing.

Ladies, the Diamond Workout is something you can do instead of the Platinum Workout program or in addition to it—because the Platinum Workout does work great for women, trust me. Diamond is also the perfect "in case of emergency, break glass" workout whenever you need to get toned and cut fast, whether it's for a wedding or your first trip to the beach and the time comes to slip into last year's bikini. If the Ladies Love Cool James, as someone once said—oh, right; me—you'll *really* love me when you're walking down the aisle in your wedding dress looking your best ever.

Before you get started, one last thing: Light some candles when you work out, feel good about yourself, and then buy yourself some flowers at the end of the week, baby. Sign my name on the card. Oh, and get a massage.

The program lasts 4 weeks, and it goes down like this. Are you ready?

**Week 1:** We start with machine circuit training, just like the Platinum Workout program does, and if you double back to the Bronze Workout, you'll see a detailed explanation for why we like to get it on and poppin' this way. To reiterate, machines allow you to get used to the movements and to learn the reps: how to explode on the positive, control the negative, and so on. Even though we're using machines here, you can definitely overload the muscle. You'll also learn to deal with post-workout soreness because where there's muscle breakdown, there's muscle soreness.

We use all machines at first. You shouldn't be touching a free weight this week (unless you don't have access to a gym, in which case we offer free-

**LL'S MUSCLE-BUILDING & LIVE-LONGER TIP** Start off your day with oatmeal. The complex carbohydrates make it a great workout fuel, leading to muscle growth. A number of clinical studies also suggest that oatmeal eaters have lower cholesterol levels and reduced risk for coronary disease than others. Oatmeal's high fiber content certainly may boost its heart benefits.

weight alternatives). We chose exercises that any gym will have; in fact, the machines will probably be arrayed on the floor in this order in some way, form, or fashion. This first week you'll go through a whole-body circuit three times with reps ranging from 15 to 20.

**Week 2:** The first major difference you'll notice in Week 2 is that we add an extra 15 minutes of work to cardio sessions. But the intensity stays the same, so you can handle it. We also need to bump up the cardio in Week 2 in anticipation of the demands increasing sharply in Weeks 3 and 4.

The resistance training changes here, too. You'll now be splitting up your body into different training sessions instead of training head to toe every time out. Rather than circuit training, you'll be progressing through workouts in conventional straight-set fashion. We also break out the 'bells (dumbbells and barbells) for the first time this week. We don't go crazy on volume, but we want to expose you to many different things, so we're squattin', we're leg curlin', we're lungin'—you name it. The really cool thing about this week's workout is that it exposes you to a wide variety of exercises, which will surprise your muscles.

**Week 3:** The big attraction and the main event for you ladies this week is that we really zero in on your quads, hamstrings, and glutes—exactly what women love to focus on. You're not worried about having 18-inch biceps, but you *do* want tight hips, glutes, and hamstrings. Am I right?

We have you doing 4 days of cardio this week, but we incorporate interval training for some wicked fat burning. Two of those days will be long-duration, low-intensity (60 to 70 percent of your maximum heart rate) work; the other two will be

higher-intensity (80 to 85 percent) intervals. At first, just raising the incline might get you to 85 percent of your max; later, you'll really have to kick it into gear to get there.

In the gym, the weights will get a little heavier this week. For first sets, we have you select a weight that causes you to fail at that 10th rep; you should pretty much have to rack it at that point. Then you finish at a weight that'll make you fail at 20. We want you lifting your heaviest when you're the freshest.

Just because we do straight sets for your upper body this week doesn't mean your heart won't be pumping and your fat-burning furnace won't be stoked to the max. You'll be moving quickly from one exercise to the next, using free weights, burning calories, working more muscles than you would during a standard machine circuit.

Then, for upper body, you do full-on circuit training. Round 1, you do a set of dumbbell rows— bam!—and then use that same weight for a dumbbell bench press—boom!—doing a set of 10, resting only as long as it takes to get to the next exercise—bam!—and then onto shoulder presses. It gives your entire body a chance to rest after a challenging set, but you're hitting it three times. It's good stuff. You'll definitely be winded.

**Week 4:** This is a doozy, in part because you'll be doing 5 days of cardio, which makes it very difficult. Again, when you're walking down the aisle or hitting the beach, you'll thank Uncle L.

Monday—leg day—is huge! Yes, that will take you a full hour. You just got to blow and go and get through it, ladies. Tuesday, I have you do some "push-pull action" to get your opposing muscle groups working synergistically: chest, back, chest, back! This is another monster day. Wednesday is great, too; arms paired with shoulders is always a fun day. Trust me, you'll feel these workouts afterward. But it's the good kind of sore.

I'm a big believer in stretching, too. A complete woman needs a complete body, and that includes stretching. In this program you'll encounter some great cardio and do some great new exercises, but you'll also fulfill the circle with some good stretching and cooldown time.

One final word: You need to follow the Platinum diets closely if you're going to succeed. Don't succumb to eating food you shouldn't because you're in search of instant gratification. Maybe you're depressed, so you want to curl up with a cupcake and watch a movie. Or whisper sweet nothings to a half a gallon of ice cream. Making sweet love to those banana muffins.

You can't use food as a source of comfort. You've got to eat to live, not live to eat.

# Week 1 (♦):
# Whole-Body Circuit Training

- Do the weight workout listed below Monday, Wednesday, and Friday; or Tuesday, Thursday, and Saturday.
- Before each workout, warm up for 5 to 10 minutes using a treadmill, a stationary bike, or some other cardio apparatus. Jumping jacks or running in place will also do the trick.
- Perform these exercises in circuit fashion; one set of leg presses, followed immediately and without rest by one set of machine rows, and so on, until you've completed one set of every exercise consecutively. Rest 2 minutes and repeat. Continue in this fashion until you've completed three circuits total.
- Choose weights that cause you to be fatigued, but not necessarily fail, on the 20th rep. Allow

the volume and resulting blood flow to work their magic here.
- On non-weight-training days, do 30 minutes of walking or stationary cycling at low intensity (60 to 70 percent of your maximum heart rate, or MHR).
- After completing your last set of every workout, go through a stretch sequence for 5 to 10 minutes targeting low back, hamstrings, glutes, and shoulders.

| MUSCLE GROUP | EXERCISE | SETS/REPS |
|---|---|---|
| **Legs** (*Alternative:* body-weight squat) | Leg-press machine | 3/15, 15, 20 |
| **Back** (*Alternative:* pulldown) | Rowing machine | 3/15, 15, 20 |
| **Chest** (*Alternative:* dumbbell bench press) | Pressing machine | 3/15, 15, 20 |
| **Shoulders** (*Alternative:* seated dumbbell press) | Overhead-press machine | 3/15, 15, 20 |
| **Triceps** (*Alternative:* dumbbell kickback) | Triceps machine | 3/15, 15, 20 |
| **Biceps** (*Alternative:* standing barbell curl) | Biceps machine | 3/15, 15, 20 |
| **Calves** (*Alternative:* standing calf raise) | Standing calf-raise machine | 3/15, 15, 20 |
| **Abs** (*Alternative:* crunch) | Crunch machine | 2/20 |

# Week 2 (♦♦): Split-System Training

- Do the weight workouts on the days listed.
- Warm up by riding a stationary bike for 5 minutes before every weight workout.
- Perform these exercises as straight sets, doing all of the sets for one exercise before moving on to the next. Rest no more than 1 minute between sets and exercises.
- After completing your last set of every workout, go through a stretch sequence for 5 to 10 minutes, targeting low back, hamstrings, glutes, and shoulders.
- Five times this week, do 45 minutes of walking or stationary cycling at low intensity (60 to 70 percent of your MHR).

## Monday

| MUSCLE GROUP | EXERCISE | SETS/REPS |
|---|---|---|
| Legs | Leg extension (warmup) | 1/20 |
| | Smith-machine squat | 2/15 |
| | Lying leg curl | 1/12 |
| | Dumbbell lunge | 2/15 |
| | Seated calf raise | 2/20 |
| Back | Pulldown | 1/20 |
| | Seated cable row | 2/15 |
| | Dumbbell shrug | 1/15 |
| Biceps | Standing barbell curl | 2/15 |
| | Incline dumbbell curl | 1/15 |
| | Preacher curl | 1/15 |
| Abs | Crunch | 2/25 |
| | Reverse crunch | 2/25 |

## Tuesday

| MUSCLE GROUP | EXERCISE | SETS/REPS |
|---|---|---|
| Chest | Incline barbell bench press | 2/15 |
| | Dumbbell bench press | 1/15 |
| | Cable crossover | 1/15 |
| Shoulders | Seated barbell press | 2/15 |
| | Dumbbell lateral raise | 1/15 |
| | Bent-over lateral raise | 2/15 |
| Triceps | Pushdown | 2/15 |
| | Overhead dumbbell extension | 1/15 |
| | Dumbbell kickback | 2/15 |
| Abs | Crunch | 3/25 |

## Wednesday

No weights, but use this for one of your five cardio workouts this week.

## Thursday

Repeat Monday's workout.

## Friday

Repeat Tuesday's workout.

## Saturday

Repeat Wednesday's workout.

## Sunday

Rest

# Week 3 (◆◆◆): Getting Your Rear into Gear

- Warm up by riding a stationary bike for 5 minutes before every weight workout.
- If 3 sets per exercise don't wear you out, add an extra set.
- After completing your last set of every workout, go through a stretch sequence for 5 to 10 minutes targeting low back, hamstrings, glutes, and shoulders.
- Do 4 days of cardio this week. Two days should be long-duration, low-intensity work (60 to 70 percent of maximum heart rate) for 45 minutes. Two days should be interval training; for example, warm up for 5 to 10 minutes; work for 2 minutes at 80 to 85 percent of MHR; work for 3 minutes at 60 to 70 percent. Continue alternating for 45 minutes. Cool down for 5 minutes.

## Monday

| MUSCLE GROUP | EXERCISE | SETS/REPS |
| --- | --- | --- |
| Legs | Barbell squat | 3/10, 15, 20 |
| | Leg extension | 3/10, 15, 20 |
| | Dumbbell lunge | 3/10, 15, 20 |
| | Romanian deadlift | 3/10, 15, 20 |
| | Glute extension | 3/10, 15, 20 |
| | Seated calf raise | 3/10, 15, 20 |
| Abs | Hanging knee raise | 2/10 |
| | Double crunch | 2/15 |

## Tuesday

### Round 1

Rest only as long as it takes you to get from one exercise to the next.

| MUSCLE GROUP | EXERCISE | SETS/REPS |
| --- | --- | --- |
| Back | One-arm dumbbell row | 1/10 |
| Chest | Dumbbell bench press | 1/10 |
| Shoulders | Seated dumbbell press | 1/10 |
| Biceps | Standing barbell curl | 1/10 |
| Triceps | Skull-crusher | 1/10 |

Rest 1 to 2 minutes.

### Round 2

Rest only as long as it takes you to get from one exercise to the next.

| MUSCLE GROUP | EXERCISE | SETS/REPS |
| --- | --- | --- |
| Back | Seated cable row | 1/15 |
| Chest | Incline dumbbell bench press | 1/15 |
| Shoulders | Dumbbell lateral raise | 1/15 |
| Biceps | Preacher curl | 1/15 |
| Triceps | Overhead dumbbell extension | 1/15 |

Rest 1 to 2 minutes.

### Round 3

Rest only as long as it takes you to get from one exercise to the next.

| MUSCLE GROUP | EXERCISE | SETS/REPS |
| --- | --- | --- |
| Back | Pulldown | 1/20 |
| Chest | Pushup | 1/10 |
| Shoulders | Upright row | 1/20 |
| Biceps | Hammer curl | 1/20 |
| Triceps | Dumbbell kickback | 1/20 |
| Abs | Hanging knee raise | 2/15 |
| | Double crunch | 2/15 |

## Wednesday

Repeat Monday's workout.

## Thursday

Repeat Tuesday's workout.

## Friday

Repeat Monday's workout.

## Saturday

Cardio

## Sunday

Rest

# Week 4 (◆◆◆◆)

- Warm up by riding a stationary bike for 5 minutes before every weight workout.
- Perform these exercises as straight sets, completing all sets for one exercise before moving on to the next. Rest 1 to 2 minutes between sets and exercises.
- Do 5 days of cardio this week. The 1st, 3rd, and 5th days should be long-duration, low-intensity work (70 percent of MHR for 1 hour). The 2nd and 4th days should be interval training; for example, warm up for 5 to 10 minutes; work for 2 minutes at 85 percent of maximum heart rate; work for 3 minutes at 70 percent. And continue alternating for 45 minutes. Cool down for 5 minutes.
- After completing your last set of every workout, go through a stretch sequence for 5 to 10 minutes targeting low back, hamstrings, glutes, and shoulders. This helps with recuperation.

## Monday

| MUSCLE GROUP | EXERCISE | SETS/REPS |
|---|---|---|
| Legs | Barbell squat | 4/10, 12, 15, 20 |
| | Leg press | 4/10, 12, 15, 20 |
| | Leg extension | 4/10, 12, 15, 20 |
| | Stepup | 4/10, 12, 15, 20 |
| | Dumbbell lunge | 4/10, 12, 15, 20 |
| | Romanian deadlift | 4/10, 12, 15, 20 |
| | Lying leg curl | 4/10, 12, 15, 20 |
| | Seated calf raise | 4/20 |

## Tuesday

| MUSCLE GROUP | EXERCISE | SETS/REPS |
|---|---|---|
| Back | Pulldown | 4/10, 12, 15, 20 |
| Chest | Dumbbell bench press | 4/10, 12, 15, 20 |
| Back | Seated cable row | 4/10, 12, 15, 20 |
| Chest | Incline dumbbell bench press | 4/10, 12, 15, 20 |
| Back | Bent-over dumbbell row | 4/10, 12, 15, 20 |
| Chest | Incline dumbbell fly | 4/10, 12, 15, 20 |

## Wednesday

| MUSCLE GROUP | EXERCISE | SETS/REPS |
|---|---|---|
| Shoulders | Seated dumbbell press | 3/10, 10, 15 |
| Biceps | Standing barbell curl | 3/10, 10, 15 |
| Triceps | Skull-crusher | 3/10, 10, 15 |
| Shoulders | Dumbbell lateral raise | 3/10, 10, 15 |
| Biceps | Preacher curl | 3/10, 10, 15 |
| Triceps | Pushdown | 3/10, 10, 15 |

## Thursday

Repeat Monday's workout.

## Friday

Repeat Tuesday's workout.

## Saturday

Repeat Wednesday's workout.

## Sunday

Rest

Sweat for your man
**Both hands on your hips** for your man
Me and the boys is your biggest fans
Every time we see you
**we be like DAAAAAAAMN!**

—LL Cool J, **"Move Somethin'," 2004**

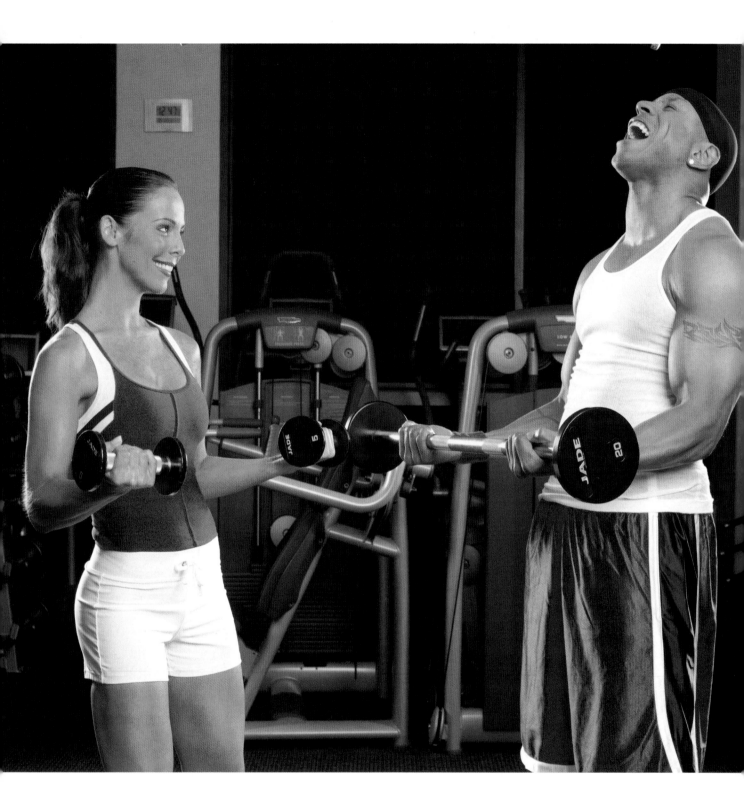

# chapter seventeen

# PHYSICAL GRAFFITI, LL COOL J' STYLE

**I**'M OBSESSED with being the best that I can be and maximizing what I am. What I'm not obsessed with is sexiness. I'm not a guy who stares into the mirror for 4 minutes, let alone hours. I'm far from that. I shave and I leave. My nails are clean because I wash my hands and take a shower, not because I'm sitting around filing them. That's the truth.

There are a lot of better-looking guys out there than me, know what I'm sayin'? I'm not gonna sit here and act like I'm the ugliest guy in the world, but what I'm not is a prima donna type who tries to be a pretty boy. That's not what I am. If a person wants to look at me as someone who's attractive, or fairly attractive, or whatever you want to call that, it would have to be in the same vein as an Oscar de

> We are all artists, creating our masterpiece with the brushstroke of each action.
>
> —L. WALKUP

la Hoya or another boxer, where the look is part of it, but it's not just about that. Like I would never be a model. No disrespect to them, but that's just not what I am.

That doesn't mean I don't have or appreciate a sense of style. Whether it's jewelry or a baseball hat or this silver chain I have attached to my belt right now, I do all kinds of stuff that's just me. For me, a lot of that comes from being raised in New York City. See, the interesting thing about my life is that I'm from the street in Queens, but in traveling around the world, I've also been exposed to the most sophisticated things it has to offer—the "finer things" in life, however you want to define those, whether it's the cigar bar over here, or the champagne over here, or the private jet, or the hotel in France and all that. But like I said, I've also been exposed to all of the sensibilities and style that come from the street. The best way to define my personal style is a marriage of that everyday, blue-collar, inner-city vibe on the one hand, with a very high-end, European upscale mind-set on the other.

Style is a completely individual thing. One reason people say I've got it is that I didn't copy anyone; I did my own thing, and I made it work for me. Not everyone could put on a Kangol hat, a tracksuit, and shell-toed Adidas sneakers and make it work, trust me. But now that you have earned platinum membership and have the body to show for it, you should also pay some attention to displaying the total package in proper fashion, from treads to threads. So bearing in mind that style is the ultimate expression of your self, and only you know what's right for you, let me hit some quick style pointers, from treads to threads.

## GETTING INTO GEAR

Ab-ercizers, iPods, bungees, Bosus—what the heck is all this stuff? The fitness marketing machine spends millions of dollars annually pitching the latest "must-have" gadget guaranteed to change your body and your life with six easy payments of $39.99! Get toned in 2 weeks . . . Get abs in 5 weeks . . . Get ripped off as soon as you pay the price for the product.

So what do you really need to buy? More often than not, not a damn thing. If you've got a pair of sneakers, access to a gym, and some heart, you'd be amazed at what you can accomplish. That being said, however, some of this gear is tight—I don't know where I'd be without my iPod, for example. But, honestly, a lot of it is bogus. So let's cut through the fat and get down to what's real.

### Lifting Gloves

**Whatzit?** Fingerless gloves made of leather, nylon, or both that can help improve your grip while saving your hands from chapping and tearing.

**Need it?** It's a personal preference. Some people like the additional hold they get; others feel that gloves interfere with their grip—or their fashion sense. Tommy don't make no lifting gloves.

### Wrist Straps

**Whatzit?** Simple cotton or neoprene straps that loop around the wrists and then around a weight to improve lifting capacity by taking the work off the forearms and hands.

**Need it?** Up for debate. Some people argue that straps enable them to lift heavier; others say they detract from grip strength and forearm development. So again, it's a personal preference. But unless you need a kung fu grip to rip spinach cans in half like Popeye, I don't see anything wrong with using some lifting straps.

### Chalk

**Whatzit?** A big white block rubbed on the hands and arms to absorb sweat and improve grip.

**Need it?** Unless you're a professional powerlifter, gymnast, or math teacher, you won't need chalk. Besides, it's really messy.

### MP3/iPod/Radio

**Whatzit?** Different machines to bring music to your ears. They're everywhere today.

**Need it?** If you're like me, music motivates and energizes your workout. Try putting together different mixes for cardio work, lifting, even stretching. And I know y'all have got my new CD on there!

### Lifting Belt

**Whatzit?** A wide, sturdy belt made of leather, neoprene, or nylon that cinches around the waist to help support the spine and core when lifting.

**Need it?** Beginners likely won't be lifting heavy

1. **Colognes:** This is a personal thing, but I like colognes that are fresh, I like colognes that smell clean. I don't like real flowery stuff—you know what I'm sayin'?

2. **Boxers versus briefs:** I like the combination boxer-briefs, 'cause it gives you support where you need it, but at the same time, it's not so tight-fitting that you feel like Superman or something. You have the Superman but with some legs.

3. **Bling:** I like jewelry a lot. Diamonds, earrings, chains, rings, you name it. I think diamonds are great. You've got to be able to carry them, though.

4. **Baseball hats:** Love 'em. Love baseball hats. I think they fit with everything. I think you can dress 'em up, dress 'em down, they're casual, they're sporty, they're functional. They keep the sun out of your eyes.

5. **Final tip:** Never wear black shoes and white socks. Now *that's* a problem.

Oh, by the way, fellas: Don't wear spandex shorts to the gym. It's *not* cool.

---

enough to need one, but a weight belt is good for people with back injuries or a history of hernias, as well as for advanced lifters who need extra support when lifting superheavy.

## Weighted Vest

**Whatzit?** Exactly what it sounds like: a vest you wear that has added weight to it. High-level athletes often use these to increase vertical leap as well as to improve speed and agility.

**Need it?** These are great, and they can be useful when you reach the Platinum level and want to mix it up a bit. Vests can increase the intensity of a cardio session or make plyometrics and speed drills harder still. Scooter loves 'em.

## Heart Rate Monitor

**Whatzit?** A two-piece system (chest band and wristwatch) that records your heartbeat. Used to monitor intensity level while training.

**Need it?** HR monitors are useful to people at all levels of fitness. They allow you to gauge your intensity level at a glance, modifying it as necessary to reach your goals. It's a great tool with which to blast off a training plateau, burn extra booty-fat, or improve sports performance.

## Swiss Ball/Bosu Ball/Balance Board

**Whatzit?** In order: a giant rubber ball, a half of a giant rubber ball on a flat platform, and a board balanced on a half of a small rubber ball. Mostly, personal trainers use these gadgets to add variety to their workouts and keep their clientele interested.

**Need it?** While it's entertaining to watch people crash and burn trying to use these things, none of them are necessary purchases. All the exercises you see people do on them can be done on the floor. The Swiss ball is more versatile than the other two, and if you've got 50 bucks burning a hole in your pocket, I'd invest in that one. But if you need to practice balancing, stand on one foot and shut your eyes. Done. And you saved 50 bucks.

## Ab Wheels, Ab Rollers, Ab-Cetera

**Whatzit?** America is obsessed with their abs, and there are tons of gadgets out there that are reputed to whittle your middle.

**Need it?** Nope. Nothing can replace crunches, core work, solid nutrition, and cardio when it comes to carving a six-pack.

## Resistance Bands/Bungees

**Whatzit?** Long rubber bands or tubing, usually with handles on either end. Used for resistance training.

**Need it?** If you travel a lot and want to work out in your hotel room, these pack easily in a suitcase and offer a viable alternative to the gym when you're in a jam. But home side, I recommend sticking to the iron. Nothing beats a solid chunk of steel when trying to buff out.

# chapter eighteen
# LIVING LARGE

Every man is the architect of his own fortune.

—SALLUST

**O**NCE YOU'VE committed to self-transformation and aced the Platinum Workout, working out becomes like a martial art. It becomes part of how you live and helps in all of your decision making. It helps when you negotiate because you're confident. It helps in everything. It clears your mind. It gives you the strength to overcome all kinds of stuff. Temptation—everything. It really helps. It *really* helps. It's a deep thing, you know?

Working out is a huge investment in yourself, and it builds up sweat equity in your body: longevity, stamina, self-confidence, and more. Because there's nothing like being able to trust yourself. That's an amazing feeling. That's how a lot of people overcome addictions and a lot of other bad stuff. That's why addictions are so depressing: because people want to be able to trust themselves. When you tell yourself that you're not going to do something, and then you do it, you feel like you can't trust yourself. Not a good feeling. Being able to trust yourself is important. *I* can trust *me*: If I say I'm going to do something, I do it. If I tell myself I'm not going to do something, I don't do it. **How about being able to trust the man in the mirror?**

I came a long way from where I used to be not only in how I looked but also in how I *think*. It all went hand in hand; it really did. It *all* gets better, not just your body. ***Today, getting in my workouts proves to me that I'm doing everything I can to win in my life. Period.*** It confirms for me that I have the courage and strength to push myself and believe in myself, and you can't buy that. It's not for sale. Not many people can look at themselves in the mirror and say, "You've done everything you can to be the best that you can be." Rarely do people make the decision to be all that they can be because it's a big decision. I remember riding on a plane several years ago, looking out the window, and just saying to myself, *You know, I'm just gonna be the best that I can. Period.*

And that's after already having enjoyed a 20-plus-year career, making more money and achieving more fame than I could have ever dreamed possible growing up in Queens. At the moment I was experiencing that epiphany, most people already would have consolidated everything, tucked the cake away, moved to Arizona, put a couple of horses on 30 acres, and just chilled out. They would be like, "Okay, I'm good. Thank you. Have a nice life."

Most people don't even get to the point where they *can* make the decision I made on that plane. Think about what it takes to get there. That's a breakthrough like splitting an atom. It's *that* deep. It's like the Manhattan Project. Once you make that decision, moving forward, everything you do in your life is based on it. Everything has changed. *You believe more, you strive to make it, you're willing to experiment, you're willing to subdue your ego, you're willing to try things that are risky, you're willing to risk looking foolish, all because you feel like you have the strength to make it happen.* Life is a series of battles, and now you've prepared to go to war.

That's not to say there aren't obstacles when you're maximizing your potential. The obstacles never end. There are always strongholds that have to be torn down. You just need the strength to deal with them. We were built to be conquerors— more than conquerors, actually. We've gone to the moon. Think about that. A lot of times the biggest obstacle I find for me is inside. There are inner obstacles and inner resistance because we're all spread so thin. We all have so many things going on. You got to dig in. You got to dig deep. *You got to be willing to cry tears of blood.* You just have to find it inside of you and be willing to go after it.

Take my new clothing company, for example. It's not easy, but it's just like working out. It all comes from the same place. There's a crucible of faith, strength, desire, ambition, perseverance, dedication, and commitment that's inside of us, and we have to tap into that thing, and nurture it, and cultivate it, and help it grow from a seed. We have to help it to blossom inside of us. That's what I attempt to do every day.

*The worst fate that can befall you is to lie on your deathbed, an old man or woman, with all your dreams standing around you, saying, "What happened? I was there for you. We could have done it."* When it's too late, don't think, *I could have worshipped more, I could have been kinder, I could have been friendlier, I could have worked harder, I could have dug deeper, I could have strived more, I could have been better.* Wow. That's something to think about, you know what I mean? That's why working out is so important—the increased energy level, the greater self-confidence, the knowledge that you're capable of doing something like that, that you can push yourself.

## Blaze Your Own Trail

Having completed the Platinum Workout plan, you can pretty much map your own route from here. Regardless of which direction you take, the key is to stay on the road and keep advancing and to continue alternating phases of higher and lower intensity training along the way. Your car won't last long if you go pedal to the metal 24/7, and neither will your body.

One thing I want to warn you about—and this applies especially to the ladies—is that as you get in shape, some important people in your life may not be as supportive as you might hope or think. In fact, they may even be threatened by your

**LL'S LIVE-LONGER TIP** Get hooked on fish. A European study of nearly half a million people found that eating a single serving of fish per day reduced colon cancer risk by 50 percent.

newfound attractiveness and self-confidence. If that goes down, that's not where you need to be. ***Eagles fly with eagles and crows fly with crows.*** A crow can't know the lofty ambitions of an eagle. If you're doing eagle business and crows are commenting, change your circle. Change your altitude. Attitude equals altitude, right? Switch up. Get rid of those people. That's not the type of a man a woman needs to be around, a guy who's telling you, "You think you're this, you think you're that." If he does, what's that say about him? There's no way he could be successful. Even if he has money, he could be a public success and a private failure.

Also, don't beat yourself up if you only got part of the way through the Platinum Workout or had some unforeseen interruptions or obstacles arise along the way. Life happens. At least you did something to better your situation; at least you're headed in the right direction now. In a weird way, learning from failure is probably one of the most exciting parts of life because when you learn from failure, you really, really, *really* increase your odds of winning. The quicker you fail, the quicker you can win. Thomas Edison—the quicker he failed at his experiments, the quicker the incandescent lightbulb was coming. Or Henry Ford—the quicker his engineers failed, the quicker the combustion engine was coming. The quicker they would fail at

## RAP SESSION: STAYIN' ALIVE

Myself, I don't have much interest in immortality, except as it can be achieved through my art, my children, and, ultimately, my relationship with God. But some longevity scientists are really pushing the envelope when it comes to how long we can live in this world before moving on to the next, and it is an interesting subject for the science fiction fan in all of us. If God blesses someone with a cure for cancer, it's scientific, but it's still a blessing to have that cure through man. As Quincy Jones once told me, "Soul with no science, and science with no soul? Neither one is effective." To find out more, I spoke with a leading expert in the fields of anti-aging science and life extension. His name is Aubrey de Grey, PhD, and he's a professor in the department of genetics at Cambridge University in England. Here's what he had to say.

**LL: Do you refer to your field of endeavor as life extension, longevity studies, or something else?**

**de Grey:** That's actually a tougher question than you would think. Colloquially, I'd refer to it as life extension, but I always point out that the important thing is the extension of healthy life because people get the mistaken idea that the goal is to keep people alive in a frail state for a long time. However,

calling it healthy life extension has its own problems because that phrase has been, if you like, hijacked by people who take the view that it's important to try to deemphasize the idea of extending total life. They think about increasing the proportion of life that's healthy without increasing the total. And that's not my idea at all. My idea is to increase healthy life indefinitely, and therefore by extension to extend total life indefinitely as well.

**LL: Have the advances in life expectancy over the past few centuries been driven by medical science, as we might expect?**

**de Grey:** Yes, but it hasn't been medical science dealing mainly with aging. In the past century, the main reason why life expectancy increased was that we stopped people from dying really young. However, if we look at death just over the past 50 years, rather than over the past 100 or 200, nearly all of the improvement in life expectancy has been the result of postponing aging and age-related diseases.

**LL: You don't see any inherent cap on human life span, right?**

**de Grey:** When people talk about a cap on human aging, they don't really disagree with me on that. What they're saying is, there's a cap on what we can achieve without intervening in aging. They say there is this inherent rate of decay that we have,

it, the closer they would get to victory. They learned from their mistakes and didn't give up.

That's where faith comes in, too: faith in yourself, and faith in a power greater than yourself, if you believe in that like I do. That's why I don't call what's happened to me luck. There was an *opportunity*, I was prepared, and God blessed me to do it. I'm only special in the sense that God blessed me to do what I'm doin', know what I'm sayin'? ***I don't really believe in luck. I have faith, and I live my life based on those principles.*** Everyone has their own outlook, but if you want to know what goes into LL's workout and into LL's life, that's part of it. It's not luck.

This book has been an opportunity to give back to people in the most important way possible, which is through the spirit. I've been able to give my spirit to you, the reader; a spirit of working hard, a spirit of believing that you can do *anything*, a faith in God, a faith in yourself. I've tried to help people take their life to the next level, and that's the ultimate charity. You can't give more than your spirit. You can give extensions of your spirit, but ultimately even if you gave a gift, it's only the spirit behind the gift that gives it value. Even if I gave you a million dollars because I had to, it wouldn't be the same as someone saying, "I love you. I want you to have this." (Even though the check would still clear—ha ha ha.) It's the attitude of giving, and that's what this

and until and unless we can fix that reasonably comprehensively, we are only going to live to some particular age. That precise age is uncertain but only slightly so. It would be around 130, maximum. However, that question simply doesn't address, and it's completely incommensurate with, the question of how long we might live if we did succeed in doing maintenance. Completely different rules of the game apply in that instance.

**LL: Scientists believe evolution occurs in leaps and bounds. Do you think that human life spans could leap forward, too?**

**de Grey:** Oh, yes, absolutely, LL. As I said earlier, it's a maintenance issue, and that means that if we can figure out how to do a reasonably comprehensive job of getting rid of the damage that inherently accumulates in our bodies over life and is eventually pathogenic and kills us, if we can do a reasonably good job—let's say, by middle age—of getting rid of that damage, then we're buying time. We're buying, say, 30 or 40 years of extra time while people are still healthy and not succumbing to age-related frailty and diseases. And 20 or 30 years is a very long time indeed in technology. So what it means is that we've got time to improve therapies and make them more comprehensive and buy us more time. This is the concept I've been calling longevity escape velocity, and it means that the transition that we'll go through will be even sharper than it might look at first sight.

**LL: That's hyped up. Where would the technological impetus for this come from—biotechnology, nanotechnology, or somewhere else entirely?**

**de Grey:** It's going to come from biotechnology because biotechnology is sufficiently far ahead at this point that we can describe in a lot of detail what remains to be done to develop sufficiently comprehensive technologies to get to the escape velocity transition. And when I say we can describe it in detail, what I mean is, we can describe it in sufficient detail that we should be able to describe the concept in a laboratory in mice, for example, within maybe only 10 years. Now, nanotechnology—in other words, nonbiological approaches to medicine—will certainly play a role in my view in the long run. But I think it's considerably further away than the biotechnological approach is. The reason it will play a part in the long run is because there are inherent limitations to what we can do with biotechnology, with what enzymes can do. That can be transcended by nanotechnology, and while we don't need to transcend those boundaries yet, we will need to in the end.

book has been about for me. Just like a concert: I give 150 zillion percent. Same here.

So what are you waiting for? Put the book down and get started if you haven't already. Do something really important. Challenge yourself. Exceed your highest expectations. Raise the bar. Go beyond what you ever dreamed possible. Take charge of your body, and in the process, take charge of your life. I went platinum; now it's your turn. That's why I've shared my story of personal transformation with the world. *This* is who I am. *This* is what I'm about.

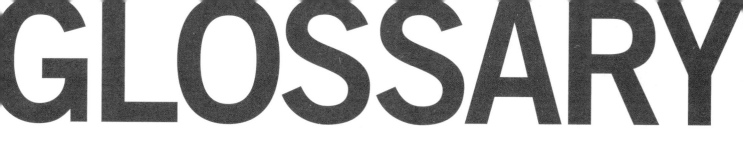

**ACTIVE REST:** Days when you don't engage in a structured workout but nonetheless remain active. An example would be riding your bike to work.

**AEROBIC EXERCISE:** Defined by the American College of Sports Medicine as "any exercise that uses large muscle groups, can be maintained continuously, and is rhythmic in nature." Most group exercise classes fall under this category.

**ANABOLIC STEROIDS:** Synthetic versions of testosterone, the male sex hormone. Used (illegally, it should be noted) by strength athletes and others to increase the body's muscle-building capabilities through increased protein synthesis, faster recovery from workouts, and other mechanisms.

**ANATOMICAL ADAPTATION:** An introductory training phase designed to make your muscles, tendons, and ligaments strong enough to train intensely in subsequent phases without injuring yourself.

**BARBELL:** A long bar with either fixed or adjustable weights on each end. Designed to be lifted by both arms.

**BIOMECHANICS:** The forces exerted by muscles and gravity on the human skeleton, used here in the context of working out.

**BLOOD PRESSURE:** The force blood exerts against the inner walls of vessels, usually expressed as a ratio. The first number refers to the pressure exerted when the heart is pushing blood; the second, to the pressure exerted when the heart is at rest.

**BODY-WEIGHT EXERCISES:** Pushups, dips, and other moves in which your own body provides the resistance.

**CALISTHENICS:** Simple exercises, such as pushups and jumping jacks, done without weights or other equipment.

**CALORIE:** The amount of energy it takes to raise 1 kilogram of water 1 degree Celsius.

**CARBOHYDRATE:** One of the three main food types, or macronutrients (protein and fat are the others), and the one the body relies upon the most heavily to satisfy its energy needs. Digestion converts these sugars and starches into glucose.

**CARDIOVASCULAR EXERCISE:** Any exercise that raises your heart rate sufficiently to make you sweat.

**CIRCUIT TRAINING:** Moving between machine exercises in a prearranged sequence with little or no rest in between.

**COMPOUND MOVEMENTS:** An exercise that requires movement at more than one joint or set of joints. The squat, for example, requires movement at the ankles, knees, and hips; the bench press, at the shoulders and elbows.

**CORE:** All the muscles of the abdominal region and the lower back, including the "deep" muscles in between them.

**CORTISOL:** A catabolic hormone that counters the anabolic effects of testosterone and growth hormone.

**DUMBBELL:** A free weight designed to be lifted by one arm.

**EXCESS POST-EXERCISE OXYGEN CONSUMPTION (EPOC):** The additional calories burned over a number of hours after completing your workout as a result of that workout.

**FAT:** One of the three main food types, or macronutrients (protein and carbohydrate are the others), which in turn comes in three main types: monounsaturated, polyunsaturated, and saturated. The most concentrated form of calories, fat provides 9 per gram, whereas protein and carbohydrate provide only 4 per gram.

**FIBER:** A noncaloric source of nutrients that is actually a form of carbohydrate.

**FLEXIBILITY TRAINING:** Those forms of exercise, such as stretching, yoga, and Pilates, designed to make muscles more pliable and therefore less prone to injury.

**FORCE:** A push or pull.

**FREE WEIGHT:** Barbells, dumbbells, and other loading apparatus not attached to a larger mechanical device; the opposite of machines.

**FREQUENCY:** The number of workouts that occur over a given period of time.

**GLYCEMIC INDEX:** A numerical scale used for foods high in carbohydrate, predicting how much that food will elevate levels of blood glucose after consumption.

**GLYCOGEN:** The stored form of carbohydrate.

**GROWTH HORMONE:** Secreted by the pituitary gland, it causes the body to grow. Reproduced synthetically and used for muscle gain and fat loss, albeit with major health risks, such as organ enlargement.

**HDL (A.K.A. GOOD) CHOLESTEROL:** The cholesterol in high-density lipoproteins. High blood levels have been correlated with reduced risk of cardiovascular disease. I call it "catfish" cholesterol.

**INTENSITY:** The amount of weight lifted. In cardio, it refers to exertion level.

**INTERVAL TRAINING:** Alternating periods of high and low intensity within the same cardiovascular workout.

**ISOMETRIC EXERCISE:** Muscle contractions that don't involve body movement—for example, flexing your biceps instead of curling a weight.

**LDL (A.K.A. BAD CHOLESTEROL):** The cholesterol in low-density lipoproteins. High blood levels have been correlated with heightened risk of cardiovascular disease. I call it "sticky" cholesterol.

**MACRONUTRIENT:** The three main food types—protein, carbohydrate, and fat—needed by the human body in large amounts. In contrast, the body needs only small amounts of micronutrients such as vitamins and minerals.

**METABOLISM:** The chemical processes inside the body whereby some substances are broken down for energy and others are synthesized for various purposes.

**OVERTRAINING:** A syndrome of symptoms resulting from inadequate recovery from exercise over an extended period of time. Contributing factors often include lack of sleep and insufficient nutritional support.

**PERIODIZATION:** Training in discrete phases designed to achieve different, albeit related, goals, including muscle growth, strength, and definition.

**PLYOMETRICS:** Exercises that emphasize the eccentric contraction phase of a movement, meaning the muscle is stretched and then contracted. Designed primarily to increase power.

**POWERLIFTING:** A strength sport comprising the squat, bench press, and deadlift. The goal is to lift as much weight as possible while meeting certain standards for form.

**PRE-EXHAUST SETS:** Tiring a muscle with an isolation movement before hitting it with a compound movement, so that stabilizer muscles don't fail before the big muscle on the compound movement, ending the set before all of the fibers in that muscle have been fatigued. For example, doing flies for chest before bench press means that your triceps likely won't give out first on the bench press.

**PROTEIN:** One of the three main food types, or macronutrients (carbohydrate and fat are the others), and the one directly responsible for muscle growth.

**RECOVERY:** The period between workouts when your body is repairing muscle tissue and replenishing energy stores.

**REP:** Performing an exercise from start to finish one time.

**RESISTANCE TRAINING:** Appling resistance to muscles in the form of free weights, machines, resistance bands, or even one's own body weight in order to build muscle size, strength, and muscular endurance.

**REST:** The downtime between sets, exercises, and workouts.

**RESTING HEART RATE:** The number of times the heart beats per minute when you're still or nearly still. The fitter you are, the lower your resting heart rate tends to be.

**SATIETY:** The feeling of satisfaction produced by eating.

**SET:** Any number of those reps (it could be 1, 10, or 100) done in one sequence.

**STABILIZERS:** Muscles that support the muscle or muscles primarily responsible for performing a lift. They vary from lift to lift.

**STRAIGHT SETS:** The conventional approach to a workout, in which all the sets of one exercise are done in succession, separated by rest periods, before moving on to the sets of the next exercise.

**STRETCHING:** Exercise whose primary purpose is to extend soft tissues, such as muscles, as far as is safely possible, in order to lengthen and strengthen them, increasing flexibility.

**SUPERSETS:** Performing sets for two different muscle groups consecutively, with no rest in between. For example, doing a set of barbell curls followed immediately by triceps pushdowns.

**SUPPLEMENTS:** Nutrients distilled from their natural state into pill, powder, or drink form. Often called dietary or nutritional supplements.

**TESTOSTERONE:** The male sex hormone, manufactured primarily in the testes.

**TRANS FAT:** Vegetable oil that has been chemically altered to make it solid and extend its shelf life. Often found in doughnuts, chips, breads, crackers, and other processed foods. Frequent consumption is increasingly being correlated with heart disease.

**VO$_2$ MAX:** The ability to consume oxygen for conversion into energy. The greater your VO$_2$ max, the higher your fitness level.

**VOLUME:** Total number of sets being done multiplied by the reps for each.

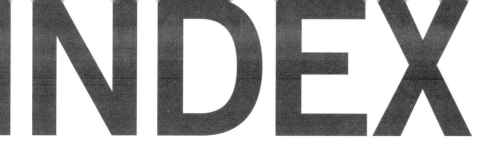

# INDEX

Boldface page references indicate photographs. Underscored references indicate boxed text.